Look
Feel
for Life
Women, Food & Exercise

april 2006

Angie,

'Read ① chapter a day'.

# Look Great
# Feel Great
# *for Life*
## Women, Food & Exercise

SUSANNE O'LEARY

Newleaf

Newleaf

an imprint of

Gill & Macmillan Ltd

Goldenbridge

Dublin 8

with associated companies throughout the world

www.gillmacmillan.ie

© Susanne O'Leary 1999

0 7171 2849 0

Illustrations by Gemma Weir

Design and print origination by

Design Image, Dublin

Printed in Malaysia


This book is typeset in 10/19pt Stone Sans

A CIP catalogue record for this book is available from the British Library.


1 3 5 4 2

To Catherine

# Contents

# PREFACE

Is there a magic formula that can make you slim, fit and healthy? As there are so many books on the subject of fitness and slimming, it would appear that there are any number of such formulas. Every year there is a new method for losing weight quickly, even stranger than that of previous years.

Fitness consultants, diet experts and even celebrities have written books selling 'the secret' for a healthy lifestyle and a slim figure. These usually contain complicated methods and strange diets that you are supposed to follow for a certain period until, just as in a fairy tale, the magic formula works, and, hey presto! A new you!

Unfortunately, this is far removed from reality. There *is* a formula for good health and fitness, but there is nothing magic about it. You can achieve good health, control your weight and improve your fitness for life. You do not have to go on diets with strange names, take pills that are hard to swallow or exercise for hours every day. There is nothing mysterious or magic about staying healthy and keeping your weight down. It just takes a certain amount of information and a willingness to make your daily life more physically active and your eating habits healthier. If you learn how the body works and how it stores (and burns) excess fat, you can apply this information to your life and transform yourself into an energetic, happy and attractive woman. It will not make you younger or change you into a different person, but it will make you feel well and in that way improve your life.

I wanted to write a book for the modern woman, be she young or old, and show her how she could change her life for the better without too much effort. I also wanted to take the bunkum out of the question of health and fitness. In my book,

I tell you about how your body works and expose the myths about weight-loss and fitness. Many people do not understand what makes you put on weight, and how to take it off and make it stay off. When you learn exactly what makes you fat, you will know how to avoid it. This book is an instruction manual of the body. If you follow the instructions, your body will work much better, and you will get years of use out of it, without it breaking down.

# ACKNOWLEDGMENTS

I would like to thank my husband Denis for his support and enthusiasm; my daughter-in-law Gemma for the wonderful illustrations; my editor Eveleen Coyle and everyone at Gill & Macmillan; and also David Cantwell for the lovely photograph on the cover.

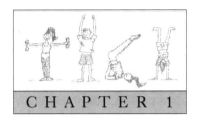

## CHAPTER 1

# LET'S GET PHYSICAL

I t is not surprising that women have no time or energy to look after their health. They are forced to forget about themselves in order to have time for everybody else. As a woman, you cannot change the demands on you, but the way you list your priorities has to change. You must put your health at the top of the list.

In this chapter, I look at the state of health of the woman of today and explain what fitness means and why it is essential to keep active. I also analyse what happened to the fitness wave of the 1970s and why most women are reluctant to exercise, especially in an organised way. I explain how you can improve your fitness without too much effort, by making it part of your everyday life. I want to remove the mystery of diet and exercise, to make it simple and enjoyable to improve your life. The secret is that there *is* no secret: you have to make it happen yourself. The rewards are many. You will feel well, have more energy to cope with the stress in your life and you will also be more confident.

## The way you live could seriously damage your health

Women are becoming more and more overweight. With every year that goes by, there are complaints from the medical world about the increase in obesity. We are constantly reminded of the dangers of an unhealthy lifestyle. In the developed

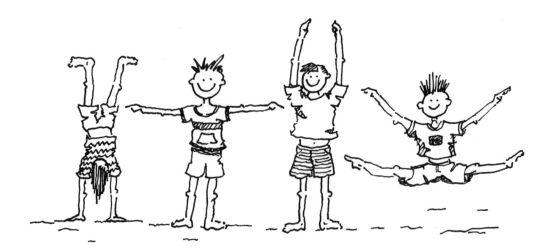

world, over 50 per cent of the adult population *are* overweight and 16 per cent of women *are* clinically obese, a figure that has doubled in ten years. The resultant health risks are too many to ignore. Seriously overweight women are two to three times more likely than slim women to die prematurely and they have an increased risk of stroke, heart disease, varicose veins, infertility and cancer of the breast, ovaries and cervix.

Most women have problems trying to keep their weight down, mainly because they do not pay enough attention to the fact that they must keep active. In principle, losing weight is simple: eat less fat and exercise more. But, in reality, it is difficult. A woman has to cope with an enormous workload every day, and not just at the office. The time you spend at work is probably the least stressful. The majority of women unwind in front of the television with something nice (and usually unhealthy) to eat after a day that would exhaust most men. Who can blame them? The problem is that, by doing so, they damage their health.

It is widely believed that most people's lifestyle has become healthier in recent years. Considering the number of health clubs and other sporting facilities that exist today, it is easy to assume that regular exercise is included in the average adult's timetable. Unfortunately, this is not true. Even though there has been a reduction in the amount of food in the modern woman's diet, it has had no effect on the problem of obesity. The composition of food has changed. Over 40 per cent of calories in the modern diet comes from fat. This is probably because turning to food for comfort is a very strong instinct. When the going gets tough, there is nothing like chocolate to cheer you up: low-fat cottage cheese just does not give you the same boost.

##  Stone-Age woman in the modern world

Why can't you eat what you like and stay slim? Put simply, because you are still built like Stone-Age woman. A woman's genetic code is still the same as it was ten thousand years ago. The human body was designed for a life of heavy physical activity: to go out into the wilderness and forage for food, to hunt and kill wild animals, to carry heavy objects, to walk great distances and to build dwelling places.

You were also designed to store energy, so that if you ran out of food you could survive until more food was available. Eating anything in sight was an instinct for survival because there might not be any food available the following day. The energy was stored in the body as fat, and also in the form of glycogen, the instantly available source of carbohydrate. Indeed, the individuals who were the best at storing energy survived the longest, so this 'talent' became a very dominant gene. Physical laziness is also an instinct inherited from primitive man. It was important to preserve energy. That is why exercise is an effort, something you have to force yourself to do.

Since the females of the species had to provide nutrition for the babies they carried, as well as for their own survival, they had to store fat very efficiently. Not only are women better at storing fat, they are also less able than men to burn it up. (Let's face it, men have it made.) Men have a greater ability to burn fat because they have more muscle, which burns fat even when not exercising. (Of course, this gives men even less excuse to put on weight!) This seems very unfair, but for primitive man, it was a great advantage. The male fat cell only had to help one person to survive, whereas the female fat cell provided food for two, mother and unborn child. This enabled the human race to survive.

However, you no longer need this way of surviving. Storing fat has become something you have to work against. The problem is that life is not as active as it once was. You never have to struggle physically to survive. Modern woman now has a very comfortable lifestyle that does not fit her Stone-Age physical make-up. Even your mother had a more physically active life than you have. Before the existence of supermarkets with their car-parking facilities, women had to go from shop to shop to get all the food shopping done. Women normally went shopping several times a week, carrying heavy bags. In this way, they got plenty of exercise just getting the food home. Housework was also physically more demanding than it is now. These days technology is there to do the work for you, and even leisure activities are becoming more and more passive. You don't need to store energy. A short trip to the supermarket soon satisfies all your needs. If your body was made for this modern life, you would have wheels on the ends of your legs, and a digestive system and metabolic rate to digest only small amounts of fuel.

##  Beware of the couch

Children have a natural instinct to be active. This instinct is discouraged at an early age. Adults often tell children to stop hopping around and to calm down. The television set is switched on to keep children quiet so they won't disturb their parents. They grow up to feel that being lively is proof of bad behaviour. The living-room couch is where most children spend their free time, either watching television or playing video games for hours on end. It is the focal point of most homes. Many people have a habit of eating while watching television, often fast food and fat-filled snacks. The sofa is becoming the place where your health is threatened the most. So, beware of the couch — it is a dangerous piece of furniture!

## The fitness wave of the 1970s and how it started

'Fitness' became a household word with the fitness boom in the late 1970s. Before then, even though exercise was considered good for you, it wasn't fashionable or sexy. After World War I, women started exercising, and physical education classes were introduced in schools. Exercise was like porridge or green vegetables: healthy but not enjoyable and not in any way fashionable. Running or other forms of exercising were something slightly eccentric people did and were not really to be admired or recommended. Exercising was done only if you had a medical condition or were training for a sport and was practised where you wouldn't be seen. Exercise clothes were unattractive and old-fashioned.

It was not until the late 1970s, when Jane Fonda made 'aerobics' the 'in' thing for women, that being fit became fashionable. Suddenly, every woman who aspired to being trendy was wearing a leotard, leg warmers and a sweat band on her head. You heard catch-phrases like 'going for the burn' and 'no pain, no gain'. A whole new way of living had started. Women were exercising not to be healthy, but to follow a fashion. Of course, many women did get very fit as a result. They discovered that you can drastically improve your figure by exercising regularly.

Jogging became popular, and tens of thousands took part in marathons in cities around the world. Marathons are still popular, but not to the same extent as a decade or so ago.

 ## What happened to the fitness wave?

The fitness industry was at its peak in the mid-1980s, but there has been a decline since then in the number of women taking exercise. It was great fun to dress up like a ballet dancer, but you had to work hard! Many women couldn't keep up the pace and gave up after a while. Another reason for the decline was that an increasing number of women started working full-time. Lack of leisure time became a problem. The industry is still doing well, but these days it seems that working out is practised by far fewer women, and then by the younger generation.

##  What is fitness?

There is a lot of talk about fitness. We are constantly reminded of the importance of keeping fit, but what does the medical profession mean by this term? Many people do not understand how fitness is connected with health.

Fitness actually refers to your heart muscle. The stronger your heart, the fitter you are. In order to make your heart strong, you have to exercise it. You make your skeletal muscles stronger by lifting weights or working against resistance. The heart works in the same way; that is, it is a muscle that must be worked to keep its strength. You can make your heart stronger only by exercising. You must push it a little every day to make this muscle improve and thus keep its efficiency. When you start to exercise, your muscles squeeze blood from your veins to your heart. Your heart has to work faster to pump extra blood around your body. The harder you exercise, the harder your heart has to work to pump oxygenated blood to the muscles, and so it becomes stronger. As you get fitter, and the heart gets accustomed to working harder, it becomes more efficient. Little by little you can cope with extra effort and your heart doesn't need to work so hard.

You will notice this mainly by the way your resting pulse is lowered. The state of your heart is generally measured by taking your pulse when you are resting. You take your pulse by placing two fingers on the inside of your wrist. When you can feel the beat, you count for fifteen seconds, and multiply the number you get by four. The fitter you are, the lower your resting pulse. A basically fit person has a resting pulse of about sixty-five to eighty beats a minute. If you have a resting pulse below sixty, you would be considered very fit indeed. If you are not fit and have a low resting pulse, your blood pressure is probably too low. In that case see your doctor. Only extremely fit people (like athletes) have a resting pulse below fifty. Your pulse rate also depends on your age. A woman over fifty who has a resting pulse of about seventy-five has an excellent level of fitness.

# Exercise is important for body and mind

An active lifestyle is essential for good health. Physical activity keeps your heart, joints and muscles in good condition. It gives you energy, boosts your immune system, helps you cope with stress, makes you feel happy and slows the ageing process.

### Take care of your heart

If you are mostly inactive, your heart gets accustomed to not working, and cannot cope with any extra effort. The heart is one of the most important organs in the body. It should be treated with respect and care. This wonderful piece of machinery will continue to work, without maintenance, for seventy years and more, if you are lucky. Heart disease is on the increase in the Western world. It is a disease of our times. It was quite rare before World War II; in fact, it was so rare that doctors in Britain had to notify the coroner of a death from a heart attack. Many heart attacks occur when an inactive person suddenly puts pressure on a heart that has never been made to work hard. There are many times in your life that you need to be able to make a little extra effort: running for the bus, putting up with stress at work, carrying heavy shopping, lifting children (a two-year-old is heavy, especially if he resists), to take just a few examples. If these things occurred several times every day, they would in themselves make your heart fit. It is the occasional and sudden demand for energy that creates the danger. If you are unfit, no matter what your age is, this extra effort puts a lot of strain on your heart, which finds it difficult and exhausting to cope.

### Work your muscles

If you don't use your muscles, they start to atrophy; that is, they shrink and become weak. Flab sets in. Your arms, stomach and bottom sag, which is not a very attractive sight. You constantly have to fight against the force of gravity as you get older. This is because of the increasing lack of elasticity in the skin. Toning your muscles helps reduce this effect.

Joints get stiff, aches and pains become more frequent, and so any activity becomes increasingly difficult. The less you do, the stiffer you get. Inactive people lose muscle fibre at the rate of 3 to 5 per cent every decade after the age of thirty. That is 30 per cent loss of muscle fibre by the age of sixty. Atrophied muscles are not a natural sign of ageing, but of inactivity. It is possible to keep a very good level of muscle tone well into old age. Remember this when you settle down to watch your favourite soap opera!

Inactivity also slows down your metabolism and leads to great problems in keeping your weight down. Toned muscles burn more calories than weak ones, even when you are not exercising. That is why it is essential to include muscle toning in your fitness routine.

### Exercise gives you energy

An active lifestyle reduces blood pressure, as it benefits the heart and the entire cardiovascular system. Being fit also gives you more energy. A fit person has more energy at five o'clock in the afternoon than an unfit person has at lunchtime. Exercising makes you feel less tired, strange as it may seem. A walk during your lunch hour or in the evening after work is very stimulating. You also sleep better if you keep fit because you are able to fall asleep more quickly and are more relaxed. All that activity makes you sleepy!

### Coping with stress

Human bodies are designed to respond physically, rather than mentally, to stressful situations. This instinctive reaction is known as the 'fight or flight' response. In times of stress, your body produces natural substances that can cause you to feel stressed or anxious. As you cannot bash somebody on the head when they annoy you, or run away when you feel threatened, the energy builds up in your body and you feel frustrated and panicky. Physical activity can burn off that energy, helping you to feel relaxed.

Many illnesses are related to stress, such as heart disease, high blood pressure and diseases of the digestive tract. Prolonged stress can weaken your immune system, making you more susceptible to minor illnesses. If you exercise, you can prevent the onset of many of these conditions, as well as giving your immune system a boost.

## Exercise relieves depression

An active life has been proven to relieve mild forms of depression because when you exercise, endorphins — some of the body's natural hormones — are released in the blood. These hormones are natural pain killers, but they also give feelings of well-being. When you exercise, your body starts to produce endorphins after about twenty minutes, making you feel wonderfully invigorated and positive. This feeling lasts a long time after you have stopped exercising. It became known as 'runners' high' when many people started jogging and taking part in marathons in the late 1970s.

## Stay active

As you grow older, it becomes even more important to keep active. Few can be unaware of the importance of exercise for women approaching the menopause. Newspapers and magazines are full of articles about this. One of the many benefits of staying active is the reduction, or even prevention, of osteoporosis, a disease that makes a person's bones grow thin and brittle, causing them to break at the slightest impact. This disease affects mainly women and is thought to be hereditary.

The older you are, the more you need regular exercise. It helps prevent thinning of bones, makes your heart and lungs healthy and reduces many diseases associated with ageing. It also increases muscle strength and may improve your balance and coordination, which can reduce the likelihood of you falling over. It helps you cope with everyday chores like carrying grocery bags, cooking and taking care of housework. Being active will help you to remain independent and not become a burden on anybody. Meals on Wheels is a long way off, if you keep active!

##  Why are so many women unfit?

Fitness is still a very popular subject in the media. Innumerable books, magazines and newspaper articles have been written about it. Many famous women have produced exercise videos, even if they are not remotely connected to sport or the fitness industry. It seems that a woman is not fulfilled as a supermodel or actress if she has not appeared in a leotard, tying herself in knots in a fitness video. The shops are full of different kinds of exercise clothes. Fitness seems easily available for most people. Why, then, is the average adult unfit? Why are our parks and woods not full of people taking exercise? Why does keeping fit seem so hard and complicated?

The fitness industry itself is largely responsible. Fitness has become a commercial gold-mine and has changed from being quite simple to a completely different concept, where methods of working out change rapidly. You have hardly started to get used to one way of getting fit, when there is something new, which is claimed to be better than anything that went before.

There is high-impact aerobics, low-impact aerobics, callanetics, step aerobics, funk, slide, dancercise and jazzercise. Some of them have to be practised with pieces of equipment, either a platform to step up and down on or a plastic sheet you lay on the floor to slide on. Sometimes you even have to hold weights in your hands as you work out, which could be highly dangerous for the badly coordinated woman. It could lead to injuries and maybe even law suits, if you dropped a weight or let it fly in someone's face. You are led to believe that this is the only way to keep fit — until something new comes along. This is misleading, since all you really need are a pair of comfortable shoes and maybe a tracksuit. Your only equipment should be your own body.

##  The problem with health clubs

A fitness club can be a very intimidating place, with its sophisticated machines, like modern torture instruments, and all those sweaty people pumping iron, with eyes bulging and muscles popping out of their T-shirts. Then there are the aerobic classes with deafening music and complicated movements. The fitness instructors themselves, be they male or female, would put you off exercise for good: tight, taut bodies in multicoloured leotards, big shoulders, tight little behinds and thighs made of steel. None of them seem to be over the age of twenty-five. They look like something from another planet; and they shout at you!

Many instructors seem to spend the whole lesson looking at themselves in the mirror, amazed by their own reflection. I suppose if you looked like that, you *would* be quite amazed. Some of them seem bored and unwilling to make sure that you do the exercises correctly. A normal couch potato, even with the best intentions of starting a fitness programme, soon realises that she will never look like them. There are often big mirrors in these clubs. Seeing your wobbly bits bobbing up and down soon puts you off, and you go home, throw away the leotards and have a bar of chocolate to cheer yourself up.

How many hours of working out would it take to be able to wear one of those garments called a 'thong' (it even sounds painful), with just a little bit of material between your buttocks? Talk about mission impossible! Be realistic and lower your aspirations. Try to accept yourself as you are, and learn to like it. The important thing is that you start to get active for the sake of your health, not just because you are upset about the way you look.

##  Health and fitness books

There is no shortage of literature on the subject of keeping fit. Most bookshops have a whole section devoted to books about health and diets. Some are meant to be handbooks, to be used as a reference when you do your daily fitness routine. Many of you probably have at least one of these gathering dust on your bookshelf. These publications are usually read once, then never picked up again. The titles are very promising and encouraging. *Get Slim and Fit Now!* one of them urges, while another tells us *How to Look and Feel Half your Age* (if only it were possible). *A Flat Stomach in Half an Hour* is a book that tries to make us believe we can achieve the impossible. Then there is *Eat What You Want and Take off Pounds* (a likely story), and *Bodyworks* (which sounds as if it has something to do with your bowels). There are many more: *Fitness for Life,* the YMCA book of exercises, and even the good old *Canadian Air Force Exercise Programme.*

Fitness books often have charts to help you calculate how much you should weigh. They have a chart for measuring your 'body mass index', replacing the traditional 'if you can pinch more than an inch' method. The 'height to weight ratio' is another formula. It should not be so scientific; you want to get fit, not do maths! The only important equation is: too much fatty food + not enough exercise = an unfit, fat body. You shouldn't have to use a calculator or a ruler, or, when all else fails, have to ask your children for help to work it out. This will not help your self-esteem (especially having to ask your children!).

##  You do not have to sweat

All the information and advice is overwhelming. You know it is 'out there', that the fitness clubs are only too delighted to take your money and make you into a lean, mean machine. The problem is that it is not really *you.* Putting on something revealing in order to follow a complicated exercise routine is not your idea of fun and relaxation. Sweating is especially unpleasant for most people. If you are not used to physical strain, getting hot and sweaty is something you want to avoid. It also totally ruins a 'good hair day'.

However, you do not *have* to sweat in order to get fit. That is the whole point of my method. I will show you how it is possible to improve your physical and mental health with very little time and effort, how you can build a fitness programme into your life without spending money on instruction, health clubs and outfits and without having to give up a lot of time. I will also show you how you can cut down on your food intake, and *maybe* start to lose weight, or maintain it, without going on a specific diet. This is *not* about achieving the perfect figure or how to be beautiful in the conventional sense. It is about normal people like you, like me, like your friends, and how to feel better. Forget about the perfect woman that fashion has decided you have to be. Concentrate on being attractive on your own terms.

Changing your lifestyle to a healthier one seems a nearly impossible task, requiring enormous amounts of hard work and sacrifice. That is why most people don't even bother to try. It is easier to stay the way you are and just put up with it. It is widely believed that if you are just slightly larger than the conventional 'norm', you are overweight. This is not true. Just to take one example; if you are 1.73 m (5 foot 8 inches) tall, you can weigh up to 70 kg (11 stone) and still not be considered overweight in the medical sense. It all depends on your lifestyle.

A big woman can be much fitter than her thinner, unfit friends if she exercises and eats in a healthy way. 'Thin' does not equal fit. Since muscles weigh more than fat, you can allow yourself to weigh in at quite a heavy weight, if you exercise regularly. In fact, you should not be too much of a slave to the weighing scales. It is best to weigh yourself once a month to keep track of your weight.

I believe that you know when you are overweight without using the scales. Try this: look down as you stand straight. Can you see your feet? No? Then you are fat! If you can see your feet, you are thin (or have big feet). If you are honest with yourself, it is not hard to figure out when it is time to take action.

Most women start fitness programmes and diets at regular intervals, often with great success. They then usually slide back to square one when they have reached their goal, stop their fitness programme and go back to their old way of living. That is not the way to go about improving your health. The secret is to change your lifestyle for good, not just long enough to lose the extra weight. It is a matter of being honest with yourself and really wanting to improve — and it is not as hard as you might think.

If you put some physical activity into your everyday life and cut fat from your diet, your health will improve very quickly. Make this a permanent change and you will never again have to bother with drastic slimming programmes in the form of boring diets and exhausting work-out routines that you will probably follow for only a short period and which will nearly always result in disappointment and a sense of failure.

##  Get up and go!

So how can you resist? Doesn't it sound really tempting to try? Why not do it for a month or two? I guarantee that you will want to keep going after that. Just try this for a start: sit up straight when you watch television instead of slouching; it is much better for your back. According to a Norwegian study, you burn sixty more calories per hour when your back is straight. That alone is a reason to straighten up. Now that wasn't too hard, was it? And no sweating! How about getting up to walk around the sofa? Feel the muscles working in your thighs and imagine how it would feel to walk for ten minutes, maybe to the corner shop to buy the paper instead of taking the car. Doesn't seem so difficult, does it? Well that is how you are going to start, little by little.

You will increase the walking to thirty minutes a day, and combine it with a light muscle-toning programme that takes only fifteen minutes, three to four times a week. You can do it without wearing special clothes, as long as you are comfortable. I will also explain how you can put more activity into your day, without changing your life very much. You must think of doing this for *you*, and nobody else — not to impress members of the opposite sex, or to make somebody else happy.

The good thing is that it is never too late to start. You can begin exercising at any age, provided you start gently. Even if you have never done anything remotely active in your life, it is still possible to change. It can transform your life, both physically and mentally. Taking up a sport, or an activity like walking, can also improve your social life, because you will meet people with the same interests. It is a great challenge to improve your lifestyle, and you will be so proud of yourself. After all, you have only one body: it cannot be exchanged if it wears out. That is why it must be handled with care. If you are pleased and comfortable with yourself, you have more to give and you are good company to others.

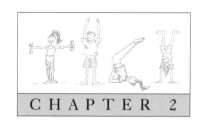

## CHAPTER 2

# NO MORE DIETS

So much has been written in the newspapers about genetic factors that many people now believe that being overweight is hereditary. It would be nice to think that it is not your fault that you became fat. Indeed, you often see families where a certain chubbiness seems to affect most family members, so you would be forgiven for believing in this theory. Recent studies show, however, that most obesity is caused by a very simple energy equation. According to the UK Medical Research Council, obesity is based on one formula: energy taken in, minus energy used up, equals the change in how much fat the body will store. In simpler terms, this means: *if you eat too much you get fat.*

Maybe it is only the inclination to overeat that is inherited. 'My mother loved ice-cream and chocolate, and so do I.' In fact, what causes weight problems within a family is most probably their eating habits and lifestyle, rather than a genetic problem.

It is also a popular belief that if you have a 'slow' metabolism, it is harder to lose weight. This has been found to be untrue for most obese persons. There are some medical conditions that would interfere with a person's metabolism, but they are rare, and very few could honestly say that they suffer from any of them.

People in the Western world are eating less per capita than they did a generation ago. Therefore, the tendency towards obesity is more about *what* people eat *and* their level of activity. In the past, people ate a larger amount of carbohydrate (starchy food). Now a large part of the energy demand is met by fat. In America, obesity is on the increase despite the health clubs, fitness equipment and personal trainers; 35 per cent of adults were defined as 'dangerously overweight' in 1994, compared to 25 per cent in 1980. And this in the country that brought us the fitness boom!

##  Grandmother's favourite recipes

We still love to eat the same type of food that our grandparents liked, although we do not work even half as hard as they did. If you look at the traditional dishes in many countries, you see that these are often very rich, covered in fatty sauces and meant to be eaten by people who were out working on a farm all day or doing other heavy physical tasks. It was all right for them to take in 3,000 calories in one sitting. They had probably burned up twice that amount in their daily activities. In addition, they only ate these rich dishes at special occasions. Their everyday diet was quite simple and consisted mostly of carbohydrates.

##  Taking it off

When you discover that you are getting fat, you try to get rid of this excess weight by going on a diet. This in itself is a good reaction; you have realised that something has to be done about what you eat. There is, however, a big problem with drastically cutting down on what you eat. The word diet in itself suggests a time limit. 'Going on a diet' means to most people sticking to a set routine for a number of weeks, until a target weight is reached, and then going back to normal eating habits. After a while their weight goes up and they start dieting again. This is the so-called 'yo-yo effect'. Most of you have probably lost and gained the same 5 to 7 kg (11 to 15 pounds) many times over.

#  The quick-loss myth

Most people want the weight off *fast*. They want it off *now*! That is why diet books promising quick weight reduction sell like hot cakes, especially just after Christmas. Sadly, there is no way you can lose a lot of fat in a short time. The articles you see in magazines of the 'I lost 20 pounds in ten days' kind are not true. It is impossible for the body to rid itself of more than about 1 kg (just over 2 pounds) of fat in a week. Anything more is water and a certain amount of muscle. Fat is a concentrated source of fuel. Your body stubbornly holds on to it for survival. If you ate nothing at all for a week, the result would still be the same.

The diet books with quick-loss promises are totally misleading. Many women spend a lot of money going from one 'miracle cure' to another. There is a fashion in diet books. One year it is *The Filmstar's Diet*, the next *The Beverly Hills Diet*. *The Airhostess Diet* of the 1970s was positively dangerous because it was based on a diet that contained only 300 calories a day, but since it was impossible to keep it up for more than a few days, nobody came to any real harm. Some fruit, such as pineapple and grapefruit, are supposed to have fat-burning ingredients.

Many people believe in 'formula' diets where a combination of some food groups and the elimination of others are said to make you get rid of weight fast. This often results in unhealthy eating habits. There is usually a considerable weight loss, but at the expense of a balanced diet. You cannot keep eating in this way for long without health problems. Also, when you reduce your intake of calories, your body automatically slows the metabolic rate. It reacts as if you are starving and tries its best to hold on to the stored energy. After only a few days on a low calorie intake, your body will no longer use up energy at its usual rate, and you will lose weight very slowly.

##  Fat-burning exercise

The combination of a low-fat diet and exercise is the most effective method to lose weight. It is important to understand how energy is stored in your body and how this energy is used. Your body stores two types of energy: glycogen and fat. Glycogen is the energy from carbohydrate in your diet. This energy is stored in the muscles to be instantly available for emergencies, for example when you need to run fast or suddenly lift a heavy weight. Fat from your diet is stored in the fat cells, which are located on the part of your body that your genes have decided they should be: on the hips and thighs of women and the stomachs of men. Fat is kept as the type of energy needed for activities sustained for a long time, for example walking, slow jogging and other types of moderate activities.

It is widely assumed that, if you work your body at a very fast rate, you burn fat more efficiently. This is not true. The type of exercise that is most effective for burning fat is moderate exercise. When you work out beyond the comfort level, you burn glycogen, not fat. When you are gasping for air, you get into oxygen debt, and the muscles need instant energy. This instant energy is glycogen. It is not until this energy store is used up that you start burning fat, which is probably about thirty minutes into your workout.

If you work at a moderate pace, however, you create the ideal conditions for the body to burn fat. As you are not short of breath, the body starts to use up the fat stores at once, without taking up any glycogen. You are unlikely to be able to keep up high-intensity exercise for very long, whereas moderate exercise can be sustained for a long period by a healthy person. Walking, cycling, swimming and rowing are good ways to get this effect, provided you do them for thirty minutes without stopping. Fitness experts call this 'LSD', 'long, slow distance'.

## Only fat makes you fat

In his book *Fitness and Health* (only available in Swedish), Professor Per-Olof Astrand explains the findings of a recent study on how the human body stores different types of energy. He discovered that it is not the amount of calories consumed that is important, but where they come from. Carbohydrate in your diet is not made into fat. These calories are stored in the muscles and liver, used as instant energy and burned off if there is an excess. Pure protein is not turned into fat either. In short, if your fat intake is low, you cannot get fat. A person who eats only fruit, vegetables, skim milk and fat-free bread can eat huge quantities without putting on an ounce. Thin people who seem to be able to eat large amounts probably have an extremely low fat intake.

 ## What is cholesterol?

Cholesterol is a waxy, fat-like substance found in every cell in the body. It is used to help digest fats, strengthen cell membranes and make hormones. Although cholesterol serves many important functions, too much cholesterol in the blood can be dangerous. The bloodstream transports cholesterol throughout the body by special carriers called lipoproteins. The two major lipoproteins are low-density lipoproteins (LDL) and high-density lipoproteins (HDL).

The 'bad' cholesterol is LDL. When there is too much of this cholesterol in your body, it can cause fatty deposits to build up on the inside of your arteries, like sludge in a pipe. The heart muscle gets its supply of blood through the coronary arteries. A build-up of fatty deposits leaves little room for the oxygenated blood to flow to your heart. Without sufficient oxygenated blood, the heart cannot function properly.

The 'good' cholesterol is HDL. It helps remove the 'bad' LDL from your blood by carrying it to the liver, where it is metabolised. It is beneficial to have high levels of HDL in the blood. Regular exercise increases the 'good' cholesterol.

High cholesterol is partly genetic and partly due to your diet. If you have a family history of heart disease or high cholesterol, it is particularly important to pay attention to your diet and level of physical activity. Studies in America show that a low-fat diet reduces cholesterol only if it is combined with exercise. Smoking is particularly harmful in this context, because it constricts blood vessels, elevates blood pressure, and raises the 'bad' cholesterol.

#  Good and bad fat

Fat provides you with calories, helps you to absorb certain vitamins, gives aroma and flavour to your food and is necessary for normal body functioning, so you should not eliminate it from your diet. But you should eat the *right* fats. It is a matter of learning the difference between the many kinds of fat in your food.

### Harmful fat

The type of fat that is the biggest risk to your health is saturated fat (found in dairy products and meat). It raises the 'bad' cholesterol and increases the risk of heart disease. The worst fat of all is called 'trans fat' (found in margarine, commercially baked biscuits, cakes, pies and bread), which is vegetable oil that is chemically hardened by the addition of hydrogen. The oil becomes steadily more saturated during the process and turns into a fat even more harmful than saturates. Look out for the term 'hydrogenated vegetable oil' on labels.

### Healthy fat

The good fats are mono- and poly-unsaturated oils (like olive and rape-seed oil) and omega-three oils (found in fatty fish). They are beneficial to your health, as they lower LDL and raise HDL. Oily fish, such as salmon, herring, sardines and mackerel, should be eaten at least once a week. Heart disease is practically unknown among the Eskimos who eat oily fish daily.

All fats are high in calories and cause an equal amount of weight gain. If you want to lose weight, you should cut down drastically on saturated fat and use mono- and poly-unsaturated fat sparingly. If you do not have a weight problem, just cut out saturated fat and switch to the other types. A maximum of 25 per cent of your diet should be fat. A meal high in fat will make you gain weight faster than if you eat the same amount of calories in carbohydrates. Fat is immediately stored in the body (usually where you least want it), whereas carbohydrates are used up very quickly. 'A minute on your lips, forever on your hips', is a good slogan to remember when it comes to fat.

The Mediterranean diet is often mentioned as an example of a healthy diet. The types of foods eaten in countries like Italy, Spain and Greece are indeed beneficial to the heart, but it is important to remember that many of these dishes contain a lot of olive oil and are thus high in calories from fat. It is, of course, the healthy kind, but the body will add it to its fat stores. It will make you fat without damaging your heart. Heart disease is not as common in southern European countries as it is in northern Europe, but many of their inhabitants are overweight. In order to benefit from such a diet, you have to reduce the amount of oil in the recipes.

##  Hidden fat that can surprise you

If you are trying to lower the amount of fat in your diet, you have probably already changed from high-fat dairy products to the low variety, and from butter to low-fat spreads. You should aim at a daily fat count of no more than 50 g (1.75 ounces). There can be a lot of fat in foods that may seem quite harmless. The foods listed below all contain saturated fats. The amount of fat (of the saturated kind) in just a small amount of any of these is staggering.

~ 1 large pork sausage, 13 g of fat

~ 1 small pork pie, weighing 140 g, 39 g of fat

~ 2 thin slices of salami, 11 g of fat

~ 1 tablespoon of whipped cream, 9 g of fat

~ 1 tablespoon of mayonnaise, 10 g of fat

~ 1 'Big Mac' hamburger, 28 g of fat

~ 1 bag of crisps, 9 g of fat

~ 1 small (60 g) bar of chocolate, 18 g of fat

~ 1 can of mushroom soup, 11 g of fat

~ 1 small pizza, 28 g of fat

~ 1 handful of peanuts, 12 g of fat

~ 1 slice of cream cake, 6.5 g of fat

You can see how easy it is to consume quite a large amount of fat without even noticing it and while not eating very much. If your lunch consisted of a bag of crisps, one small pork pie and a small bar of chocolate, you would have clocked up an amazing 66 g of fat, which is a lot more than you should eat during the entire day! If you went in to the pub for a drink on the way home and had a handful of peanuts as well, you would add another 12 g of fat before you even sat down to eat your evening meal.

In contrast, on a low-fat diet you can eat big meals while still keeping your fat consumption very low. A low-fat day could consist of the following:

**Breakfast**
Two weetabix with one cup of skim milk, a banana and half a grapefruit.

**Lunch**
A sandwich made with two slices of wholewheat bread, water-packed tuna, one tomato, two teaspoons of low-calorie mayonnaise, one low-fat yogurt and one orange.

**Dinner**
Two pieces of skinless chicken breast, baked in the oven or poached, one baked potato, one cup of yogurt dressing, one cup of broccoli, one cup of lettuce with low-fat dressing, half a melon and two glasses of wine. You can in addition eat as much fruit as you want.

With this type of diet, only about 8 per cent of the calories come from fat. You can eat a lot of food, without putting on an ounce. You do not have to count calories, only the fat. A low-fat diet also supplies you with many vitamins and a lot of dietary fibre.

##  Reading the labels

The most important item to bring when you go shopping for food (apart from money) is a pair of reading glasses. You could also have a stiff drink before you go; shopping these days is stressful. The children play up, the trolley gets stuck and *you have to read the labels*! Nowadays you practically need a degree in nutrition to figure out how to feed your family in a healthy way. It is important to read the labels on everything you buy. Food manufacturers are required to list their ingredients in descending order. The higher up the list an ingredient is, the more there is of it in the food. The different types of fat also have to be listed. It can be depressing to find that your favourite treat contains large amounts of saturated fats, additives and sugar, but it is useful when you are trying to eat in a more healthy way.

Some manufacturers claim that their food has a defined nutritional value. These claims can be deceptive; a reduced-calorie food could still be high in sodium, a low-fat food high in sugar. Various fats and sugar can occur several times throughout the lists of ingredients. If the first ingredient is not sugar or fat, it does not necessarily mean it is a healthy food.

### ❭ Low-fat foods

There are many products on the market that are labelled as 'low-fat', 'low cholesterol' or 'light'. It is natural to think that these foods can be consumed in unlimited quantities. This is not so. These products *do* contain fat, and often a lot of sugar. Even though the fat content is lower than the traditional variety, it is still present. Low-fat biscuits contain about 60 calories per biscuit, half of which come from fat. 'Low cholesterol' in big print hides saturated fat content in small print. Indeed, many low-fat foods contain less fat than their full-fat equivalent, but the fat is saturated. 'Light' can also mean less colour; olive oil labelled as 'light' is just lighter in colour and has the same amount of fat as the darker kind.

Sometimes fat content is listed 'per serving'. This 'serving' can be very small. 'Reduced fat' is another term that is highly deceptive. Foods that are normally cooked in a large amount of fat (like crisps) still have to be cooked this way, so there is still a lot of fat present. 'Reduced fat' only means less fat than before, but since you do not know how much this was, how can you know what the end result is? It is better to wean yourself off things like biscuits and crisps and find something else (like fruit and vegetables) to take their place. Labels for 'low-fat' spreads are particularly misleading. Spreads are exempt from the guidelines for low-fat claims. A 'low-fat' spread could be 40 per cent fat. That makes it much lower in fat than butter or margarine, but still a high-fat food relative to others.

High-fat foods are more honest. What you see is what you get (fat), so you know that you must avoid them. The same applies to sugar substitutes. It is better to get used to taking tea and coffee without sugar than using sweeteners. There are no sweeteners that taste exactly like sugar. The taste is always a bit artificial.

## ❯ Food additives

Many foods are now 'enhanced' by additives. They are supposed to improve the colour, taste and consistency of what we eat. Strawberry ice-cream would be grey if it was not artificially coloured; so would shrimps. Food is coloured to look attractive, and the consumer has become used to this. If strawberry ice-cream *was* grey, you probably would not like it as much. Food additives can be both 'natural' and synthetic. They all have E numbers, which means they have been approved for use in EU countries. How is the poor consumer supposed to know what all these numbers mean? Some people are allergic to additives in food, for example E 220-28 (sulphur dioxide and sulphates). Usually found in dried fruit, desiccated coconut, fruit pie fillings, relishes and wine, these can trigger allergic reactions, especially in asthma sufferers. Another additive is tartrazine (E 102), which is found in yellow-coloured sweets, squashes and other soft drinks. This may also cause allergic reactions and hyperactivity in sensitive children.

Labelling food to inform the consumer of content and sell-by dates is very useful, but it would be better to remove many of the artificial ingredients. It is up to the consumer to show manufacturers that these foods are not desirable by not buying them and switching to more natural foods. Eating more food without additives does not have to increase your supermarket bill. It could mean, however, that you have to spend more time preparing your meals, resulting in better tasting food of higher nutritional value. Is that not worth the extra effort?

##  The advantage of carbohydrate

Eliminating the unhealthy foods from your diet will not make you go hungry. Carbohydrates in the form of fruit, vegetables and starch can be eaten in large quantities. If you eat as much of these foods as you are supposed to, in order to fill the daily requirement of your body, you will not feel starved. As fruit and vegetables contain no fat, you can eat as much of them as you like.

There are three types of carbohydrate: sugar, starch and fibres. Sugar gives a lot of energy but no vitamins or minerals. Starch, which is found in potatoes, pasta, rice and bread, is a better source of energy than sugar. Fibres, which are found in fruit, vegetables and starchy foods, don't give as much energy but are healthy in other ways. A diet high in fibre reduces the risk of heart disease and bowel cancer. Fruit and vegetables also contain many vitamins and minerals essential for good health. It is important to keep your blood sugar high at all times so that you will not be tempted to reach for fast food and snacks that have a high content of fat and sugar.

A good breakfast high in carbohydrates is the best way to start the day. Unfortunately, many people manage only a slice of toast and a quick gulp of coffee before rushing out the door. Some even skip breakfast altogether. It is not surprising that these people head for the sweet machine or cake shop at eleven o'clock. Your blood sugar is low after the night's fast. You need to raise it, and to replenish your energy stores for the day to come. Eggs and milk are excellent sources of protein. The egg (only one) should be poached or boiled and the milk low-fat. Unrefined cereals and wholemeal bread provide slow-acting carbohydrates. Cereals low in sugar are the best (check the labels). The traditional fried breakfast should be a thing of the past. A plate of the conventional 'fry' contains an average of 800 calories, and an artery-clogging 61 g (over 2 ounces) of fat! It used to be said that you should 'breakfast like a king, lunch like a prince, dine like a pauper'. It is still a good rule to follow.

##  Roast it, poach it, steam it, grill it, but don't fry it

So, you have come home from the shop with your low-fat fish, skinless chicken and lean meat. Well done, a thousand brownie points! Now you have to cook it without adding to the fat count. Good nutrition is about *how* you cook as well as *what* you buy. Fat is added to food during cooking to add taste, to seal in moisture and to make sure that most of the food does not stay stuck to your pan. With the right technique and utensils, you can have the same result without adding fat.

Dry roasting, either in the oven or in a non-stick frying pan, is one method of cooking without fat. A good Teflon-coated frying pan is ideal for cooking meat. Even lean meat has enough natural fat to be cooked like this. The empty pan should be heated for two minutes before the meat is added. If you find that the meat still tends to stick, use a little spray-on oil. Roasting in the oven is even better. Chicken, peppers, squash, root vegetables and potatoes can be cooked in this way. Use a non-stick dish and season vegetables with salt before putting them in, to help the juices escape. The temperature should be medium (gas mark 6/400°F/200°C).

Poaching and steaming are other methods suitable for cooking fish and vegetables. You can buy saucepans that are specially made for steaming. For poaching, you can use any saucepan. Poaching is particularly good, because you can poach the food in various stocks with added herbs.

Meat, oily fish and chicken are all delicious if grilled. They can be prepared under an oven grill, in a grill pan or on an outdoor barbecue. The food can be marinated in spices and herbs before cooking and served with salads and baked potatoes.

The microwave oven is another very useful appliance for cooking without fat. Fish cooks beautifully in the microwave. So do most vegetables and potatoes. The microwave is a wonderful invention for the busy life we all have these days. It is a good investment for both healthy eating and convenience.

##  Low-fat recipes

There are many cookery books which contain low-fat recipes. They can be found in the cookery book section in most bookshops. My particular favourites are the books produced by the Weight Watchers' association. They are full of wonderful recipes for dishes that you wouldn't be embarrassed to serve even at dinner parties. If you like cooking, you will enjoy preparing dishes from these books. They are readily available in bookshops and easy to find, as they are always labelled with the Weight Watchers' logo.

*The Fatfield Recipe Book* by Sally Ann Voak (published by Michael O'Mara Books Limited) is another book I have found useful. It was published in 1992 as a follow-up to a programme about slimming on the BBC. The recipes are simple to follow and the dishes really tasty. There are also many tips on how to replace traditional snacks, sauces and dressings with fat-free alternatives.

Learning how to prepare meals with little added fat is the best way to make eating both healthy and enjoyable. You do not have to sacrifice taste in order to be healthy. Cooking like this is difficult at first, but when you get used to it, you will wonder how you could possibly have liked so much fat before. You are more likely to stick to healthy eating if the food tastes good. Boring meals will not tempt you for long.

##  A healthy diet

The main rules of a healthy diet are:

~ Reduce fat from your diet.

~ Eat more fruit and vegetables.

~ Increase your intake of carbohydrates, for example bread, potatoes and pasta.

~ Avoid the three chs: chocolate, cheese and chips.

It is quite hard in the beginning and you will miss your favourite foods. If you like cooking, it becomes quite a challenge to try to make what is healthy taste delicious. There are so many low-fat alternatives available that with a little imagination you will soon get used to a different way of eating without the feeling of too much sacrifice. It is a matter of re-educating your tastebuds and learning to like tastes and textures other than fat. The reward will be a considerable weight loss and the end to worries about getting fat.

##  Alcohol and women

A glass or two of wine with your meal (but no more) is allowed and even considered beneficial to your health. Drinking more than two 'units' (one 'unit' is one helping of an alcoholic drink: one glass of beer or wine, or one small shot of whiskey) a day is not recommended because of the health risk it carries. Women have smaller livers and weigh less than men, which means that smaller amounts of alcohol affect them more. Women also have lower levels of the enzyme that breaks down alcohol in the gut and a lower proportion of water to body fat. This means that alcohol is more concentrated in a woman's body. As a result, drinking more than the recommended amounts of alcohol is likely to do you harm.

Myths and truths about dieting

| Myth | Truth |
|------|-------|
| Eating late at night makes you fat. | It does not matter when you eat. It is your *total* fat intake that counts. |
| All calories count. | Calories from fat are most likely to be stored as fat. Calories from carbohydrates will be used up by your muscles very quickly. |
| Health foods are slimming. | Some 'health foods' contain more fat and sugar than ordinary foods. (Read the labels.) |
| Drinking a lot of water helps you lose weight. | Water may make you feel full, but not for long. Your stomach can tell whether it is full of water or food. Water can not stop you from absorbing calories from fat. |
| Combining certain foods helps you lose weight. | Some people lose weight because they eat less for a while. Food-combining does not make the body store less fat. |
| You can spot-reduce fat. | You always lose weight the same way; first from your stomach, then from your face and between the shoulder blades, and finally from your hips and thighs. |
| Grapefruit dissolves fat. | No it does not. (Wouldn't it be wonderful if it did!) |

 It is all in the mind

The only person who can change the way you eat is *you*. Nobody can do it for you. It can only happen if you really want it to. It is all very well to understand and agree to good sense, but you have to be truly committed. This is my own experience. I was once overweight and aware that I had to do something about it. It took me quite a long time to get going. I was not used to having to worry about what I ate, because I had always been slim. The food we were served in my family home was healthy. I also took quite a lot of exercise as a teenager, since my hobbies were horse riding, skiing and dancing. I walked to school like all my friends (nobody was driven to school then). In the summertime I cycled and swam daily. I had a physically active life without even thinking about it.

This all changed when I got married and had children. I stopped exercising while I was pregnant (in those days doctors didn't recommend exercise during pregnancy). When the children were small, I stayed at home eating chocolates while I watched them play. It was difficult to get out to do anything active and I ate to relieve boredom. I was soon both fat and depressed.

In the end, I couldn't stand feeling like this anymore. I got a babysitter, joined an exercise class and stopped pigging out in front of the television. In four months, I had lost 22 pounds and was fit again. This was more than twenty years ago, and I have not put on weight since (apart from a pound or two as a result of occasional festivities). The reason why I changed my lifestyle was not that I wanted to be thin and fashionable. It had nothing to do with wanting to look in a particular way. I just felt unhealthy and tired. I knew that I should be feeling well and energetic, since I was young and didn't suffer from any diseases.

It was wonderful to take charge of my life and improve my health. It was a boost to my self-esteem. The fact that I looked better with a trimmer figure and good posture had a lot to do with it, I must admit. I discovered that a healthy diet, such as the one I have described in this chapter, gives you energy. It is the simplest way to get fit and healthy. You don't have to count calories or weigh your food. It is a matter of remembering one rule: *low fat*. That's it!

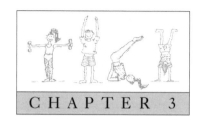

## CHAPTER 3

# BODY ANGUISH

Y ou might think that the subject of beauty has nothing to do with fitness and health. On the contrary, it has *everything* to do with it. It is often the quest for beauty that makes women take up a sport or start a fitness programme. This is also the reason many women do not exercise. They feel they would never come even close to looking like the models they see in the magazines and on television. They often feel awkward about joining keep-fit classes because they are embarrassed about how they look. Some women also give up exercise after a while, when the anticipated miracle of a perfect body does not materialise. It is a pity that women cannot accept themselves as they are. Many women have low self-esteem because they do not understand that *everybody* has good and bad points.

Women have always pursued the ambition of looking like the ideal that is fashionable for their particular period in time. In this chapter, I will analyse the problems women have with trying, and often failing, to fit this ideal. The concepts of beauty reflect political, social, economic, technological and medical developments in the world. The last six centuries have seen an ever-changing image of what is the ideal way to look. Throughout history, women have been prepared to suffer for their beauty.

## Ideals of the past

During the Elizabethan period, women wanted to look like their queen. Ladies at the court dyed their hair red and plucked their eyebrows and hairline. They used white make-up made of lead and mercury. This was highly dangerous because these ingredients could get into their bloodstream and actually kill them. Women wore tight corsets which were uncomfortable and caused health problems.

During the seventeenth and eighteenth centuries, fashion was still very much dictated by the royal courts. The ideal shape of a woman was what would today be considered obese. Just look at women in the paintings by Rubens (1577-1640): voluptuous women seemingly proud of their feminine curves. The ideal woman of that time was very different from the streamlined career woman we so admire today. A fashionable lady's clothes were cumbersome and difficult to move in. Dresses were structured with panniers underneath, extending the hips on either side, reaching enormous proportions. Elaborate wigs rose to immense heights, making it difficult for the wearer to go through doorways and enter carriages.

In the early nineteenth century, there was a short period when fashion was more natural. During the regency period, the ideal of beauty was inspired by ancient Greece, particularly by Greek statues. A slim figure was beginning to emerge as the ideal shape to fit into the body-hugging, flimsy dresses. This 'natural' look was difficult to achieve for the more amply built ladies. Those who were not naturally slim had to wear tight corsets.

During the Victorian era, women's clothes became more rigid with crinolines and the still tightly laced corsets. (No wonder women were always 'swooning' in those days.) Later in the nineteenth century, skirts became more narrow and the bustle was used to emphasise a woman's buttocks.

The years after World War I saw a major change in society. Women, who during the war had been doing traditionally male jobs, discovered the liberation of wearing more comfortable clothes, even trousers. In the 1920s, there was a huge change in the way women dressed. They cropped their hair and wore short skirts, waistless dresses and trousers. Men and women looked more similar than ever before, both in the shape of their bodies and in their hairstyles. Cosmetics were mass produced, so the fashionable women of all classes wore make-up. Royalty no longer dictated fashion: now it was film stars and other celebrities. The French designer Coco Chanel made it acceptable to be suntanned. (Imagine, we could all have smooth skin well into our fifties and sixties, if it hadn't been for her.) When rich people began to take their holidays on the French Riviera, a suntan became a sign of affluence. The modern woman was beginning to emerge.

Ever since the 1920s, there have been swift changes in fashion and the ideal image of beauty. The hour-glass figure was very much the thing in the 1950s. We have only to look at the films of the period to see that the female stars were much more strongly built than they are now. This was the ideal until the late 1950s, when Audrey Hepburn was at the height of her career and the malnourished look was beginning to become fashionable. Then along came Twiggy, the very first supermodel, who created a look that everybody tried to copy. She was waif-like, even on the verge of being skeletal.

Suddenly, women were supposed to look like a stick insect. This was impossible for most women. Many young girls spent all their teenage years attempting to be terribly thin with no shape at all. Exercise was not yet considered as a method to alter their figure, so women had to drastically reduce the calories in their diet. As a result, many young women were eating barely enough to keep them alive. They were very unfit and probably unhealthy as well.

This trend lasted well into the 1970s, until the start of the fitness wave with Jane Fonda at the end of that decade. Women realised that it was attractive to have a fit and healthy body. It was considered quite acceptable, even desirable, for women to have well-defined muscles. They started working out with weights, something that had been a completely male domain before. Many women discovered that exercise could give them a good figure. They became addicted to working out.

Unfortunately, the 1990s saw the return of the very thin woman and there was a decline in the number of women taking part in fitness classes. These days, the models on the catwalks are mostly girls in their teens, making it impossible for a mature woman to keep up with the ideal of today.

##  Sugar and spice

It must be a natural thing for females to think that they can be loved only for their looks. The Barbie doll is one example of how for decades girls were conditioned to think that long legs, slim hips and blonde hair are the ultimate in beauty.

In the past, a woman was always judged first by her appearance. She could be the most successful person in the world, the most intelligent and skilled president of her country, a brain surgeon or a nuclear scientist. But if she had bad legs or a less than attractive face, she was criticised for this, and her skills were considered less important. If she was stunningly beautiful, on the other hand, she had to prove she had qualities other than her looks. A beautiful woman was always thought to be less than moderately intelligent. These days, fortunately, women do not have to live up to the ideal of being attractive above all else. Women are now judged more on their performance than on their looks. There is still a tendency, however, to criticise a woman if she does not dress fashionably or is not well groomed, even if she has achieved great things. Let us hope that this trend will disappear in the future!

It is reassuring that the shape of the Barbie doll changed in 1998. Her breasts are now smaller, her waist (slightly) thicker and she also comes as a brunette. (I bet she has no cellulite on her thighs though: that would make her *too* real!) Hopefully, this transformation will help girls realise that the ultimate goal in a woman's life is not being pretty.

Men, on the other hand, do not have to live under the pressure of having to be handsome. You never hear anybody assume that a handsome man is stupid. It is amazing that many fat, bald, short or otherwise unattractive men have women throwing themselves at them. When men age, they grow in wisdom and experience. Young women find them interesting. When women age, they just grow old!

##  Happiness is being a size ten

I have discovered, after many years of looking at people's bodies in my fitness classes, that no two people look the same. There are as many shapes as there are fingerprints. Not one body resembles another. Despite this, most women aspire to be one particular shape.

'I must lose ten pounds to get into *that* dress.' 'If I don't go on a diet I'll look hideous at the beach.' You say this to yourself all the time. Many women equate small dress size with happiness. 'If I could only be a size ten', they say. I find this very strange, since nobody can actually see the labels inside your clothes.

The main cause of eating disorders is trying desperately to fit into an ideal image created by fashion. It is a way of controlling your life and how you are accepted. If you have nothing else to impress your friends with, you can at least prove that you are able to be thin. What most women want to be is *thin*. The nicest thing you can say to someone is: 'Have you lost weight?' You think you can be admired and loved only if you are as near as possible to this ideal. The problem is not that the ideal is a thin shape, but that there is an ideal at all. Many women fall into this trap. Indeed, you spend most of your adult life feeling rather unhappy with your body. As you grow older, you have the added pressure of having to look young!

If you look at the animal world, you discover that there are many different shapes within the same species. A greyhound could never be a Labrador, a beautiful big shire horse could not be turned into an Arab horse or a Shetland pony. It is the way they are made, and you accept that. It seems natural and normal, and you admire each one for its particular characteristics. With humans, why should it not be the same? We are all different, and every type of person has his or her charm. You can blame your parents, or nature, but you are stuck with your shape. You all have good points and bad, so try to emphasise the good ones and cover up the bad.

Everybody has some sort of talent. It could be for sports, gardening, cooking, languages or something very creative, none of which has anything to do with the size of your hips! Take your friends for instance. Do you like them because they are slim and perfect? Of course not! Most people's friends come in all sizes. You like them because they are good company, supportive, kind and fun to be with. They probably like you for the same reasons. Wouldn't it be boring to surround yourself with slim, perfect people, whose only interest was their looks?

You must try to be an individual. You should recognise the shape you are and bloom within it. Every shape is lovely in its own way and it is only within that frame that you can improve. You cannot change your basic shape or build. It is time for women to stop paying attention to what the media (and the businessmen in the fashion industry) dictate and start recognising what really matters: being healthy, feeling well and being happy with yourself.

##  What is a woman?

Is your waist quite slim? Do you go 'out' at the hips? Congratulations, you are a woman! A rather nice male Italian friend once said, when I complained about my shape: 'You are a woman! Why do you want to look like a boy?' Indeed, women in southern European countries are more accepting of their womanly shapes; they are not afraid of wearing tight skirts with a belt showing off their waists and their hips. Maybe that is why men consider them so sexy! The obsession with having slim hips and thighs, like a boy, is quite strange really. It is about time women started realising that a feminine body is nothing to be ashamed of.

The women's magazines aimed at the twenty-five to forty age group seem to ignore the reality of women's lives. Pregnancy and childbirth are the life experiences that will most profoundly affect a woman's body, yet you never see these mentioned in the articles that advise you how to achieve the perfect figure. There are also many articles about sex (this apparently increases the sales figures). You would be forgiven for thinking that your life is not normal if you don't have sex at least twice a day with different partners (this would greatly improve your fitness). The women in these magazines bear little resemblance to real women.

#  Typecasting

The human body does not store fat in one universal layer, but concentrates it on one area. Where this area is depends on your sex and your genes. Men generally store their fat around the stomach, while most women have theirs on the hips and thighs. Some women, however, store fat a bit like men, above the belt. It depends on your body type. Storing fat around the hips and thighs is a way of protecting a woman's reproductive organs. This is the healthiest body type. Fat around the lower area threatens your health less than if you have fat above your waist. Fat above the waist is constantly being built up and broken down, so fat products are released into the bloodstream where they may affect the heart and the liver.

What is your particular shape? In the 1940s, an American doctor, William Sheldon, categorised bodies according to three basic types: Endomorph, Ectomorph and Mesomorph.

### The Endomorph

The Endomorph has a rounded body, narrow shoulders, small and rounded breasts, a pronounced waist and wide hips — what we call 'the pear'. This is the most common female shape. Fat is stored on the hips, thighs and lower stomach. Why isn't this the type of body all women want? It is a shame, because if it was it would save a lot of heartache and frustration.

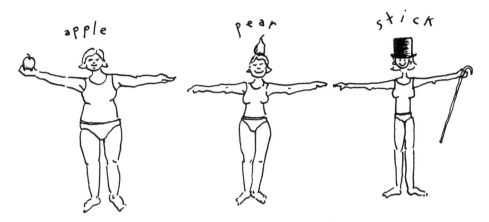

### The Ectomorph

The Ectomorph is slender, small-boned and stores little body fat — the envy of most women. Ectomorphs are angular in their shape and often wish they had more curves. They are the frail, waif-like kind that became so fashionable with Twiggy. Kate Moss is her 1990s equivalent. If you are either one of the other body types, you could never come even close to looking like these women, and that is the crux of the problem today.

### The Mesomorph

The Mesomorph has a strong, athletic shape with slim hips; when these women put on fat around the middle, they are known as 'the apple'. This shape, with its solid torso, large, rounded breasts and long slender legs, became most desired by women in the 1980s when the fitness boom was at its height. The athletic-looking woman, who proved with her strong and slightly male shape that she was extremely fit, corresponded with the sporty trend of that time. Women's clothes of that period had big shoulder pads, to emphasise this shape. The Mesomorph is not, however, the healthiest body type since she is more likely to develop heart disease and high blood pressure if she puts on weight. Her body fat is concentrated around the waist and upper abdomen. The women with this type of body have to be extra careful not to gain too much weight. (This also applies to men.)

#  Body language

Your genes lay down the blueprint of how your body is shaped. Learning to like your body is the first step to better self-confidence. Look at your shape and recognise what it is. Then try to find out how to improve it. A good posture, toned muscles and a basic level of fitness will make any shape look well. If you get used to regular exercise and a healthy diet, you feel at your very best. Think of attaining what sportspeople call their 'personal best'.

Straightening up is the best thing you can do to improve your all-over look. It will also be good for your back and shoulders. Your posture is a reflection of your personality and the amount of confidence you have in yourself. It is the signal you send out to the people around you. A woman with a straight back and shoulders looks positive, confident and happy with herself. If you slouch, you look sad, timid and unhealthy. It is not, however, a matter of walking around stiffly as if you had swallowed a poker.

Stand sideways in front of a mirror, looking at yourself in profile. Now, start by relaxing your knees; don't bend them, just relax them. Then pull in your bottom to stop your back from arching. Next, pull up at the waist and let your shoulders relax. Try to get used to this position both standing and walking. It will soon become a habit and you will be amazed at how much more comfortable you will feel. Your back and shoulders will benefit and you will also improve your shape, especially if you can in addition hold in your stomach. Toning your stomach muscles makes them strong enough for you to hold your stomach in. Stomach exercises do not in themselves give you a flat stomach; you have to train yourself to hold your stomach in.

If you learn to stand with your knees slightly relaxed all the time, you will never again have a tired back from standing. Your spine will be held in the correct position merely by relaxing your knees. It is a difference of maybe half a centimetre (one-fifth of an inch) in the angle of your spine, but it can make all the difference between comfort and pain when standing. Many women stand with their weight on one leg, jutting out their hip. This is not either particularly attractive or good for your back. You will soon develop lower back pain. It is not generally known how fragile your back is and how important it is to keep it in the right position. Bad posture is what most ruins a woman's appearance. It can make a potentially beautiful woman look unattractive. How right mothers are when they tell children to straighten up!

##  Get some support

My grandmother swore by good-quality underwear. In her youth, the so-called 'foundation garments' were very important, since they were what held a woman in everywhere. When women did no exercise, they had to rely on corsets to give them the appearance of having a good figure. These days you know that exercise can trim the muscles of your own natural corset. However, age, childbirth and gravity make their mark, so sometimes it is necessary to give nature a helping hand. Although exercise is essential for your health and effective in giving you toned muscles, it is not always possible to look as trim as you would like. Women of today do not have to wear the elaborate corsets of their mother's and grandmother's time. There are lots of undergarments these days that are both comfortable and effective.

A good-quality bra is maybe the most important item in your wardrobe. The women's liberation movement in America during the 1970s urged women to burn their bras. This was silly, since a good bra is a girl's best friend. The 'low-slung' look is neither attractive nor particularly liberating. You feel much better if your bust is supported by a well-fitting bra. They are of much better quality nowadays than they used to be. The underwired variety is much more comfortable than before, and gives a great 'lift', to both your body and your morale. If you have a big bust, a sports bra is a good solution, even when you are not exercising. It both supports and slightly flattens your bust, which may make clothes fit you better and make you more comfortable.

Most department stores have assistants who are trained to fit you with the proper bra. If you have never had a professionally fitted bra, get one now! It makes a huge difference to the way your clothes fit, and it does not add to the cost of the purchase.

##  Tighten up!

Another item that is beginning to make its mark is the new type of tights, the 'control tights'. They have extra hold in their upper part and hold in your stomach, your bottom and even your thighs. They are comfortable and quite cheap. It is a great way to help you look trim, but will not in any way replace exercise. If you don't exercise, no amount of underwear will improve your health or your looks. You cannot cheat! In any case, you do not want to wear tights in the summer, when it is hot, so you have to keep your muscles toned.

Well-fitting underpants are also important. Gone are the days of the annoying condition known as 'VPL' (visible panty line); nobody should have to suffer from it these days. Also, remember to always wear clean underwear.

##  Beautiful — on your own terms

Accepting and liking yourself is not easy, but you get such a feeling of freedom and satisfaction when you do. Forget about the images of so-called perfect women. First of all, try to *feel* well. Then you will also look well. You will be truly beautiful, but on your own terms.

While it is unhealthy to be very overweight, it is equally unhealthy to constantly sacrifice your health with faddy diets, gaining and losing weight at regular intervals. You should change your goals first of all. If you can get away from the idea that it is largely your looks that decide your happiness, then you will go a long way towards having a better life. What you should do is change your lifestyle a little, take some exercise, eat what is good for you and try to eliminate the unhealthy things in your life. You don't have to dig out those leotards from the back of the wardrobe, or put on a pair of those awful bicycle shorts. (It should be against the law for anyone over the age of twelve to wear them.) There are many ways to make your daily life more active without spending time doing sports you don't enjoy.

When you get used to it, you will notice how much better you feel. It won't drastically change your life, but in some ways it will revolutionise the way you see yourself. It can only be an improvement. The difference will be the happy look in your eyes, a trimmer body and an increase in energy.

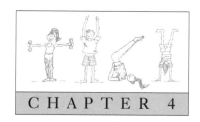

# WHEN THE GOING GETS TOUGH, YOU WANT TO EAT CHOCOLATE

Eating is the strongest human instinct and the most important activity in most people's lives. Food is also one of life's greatest pleasures. We gather around a meal with friends and family. It is a way of sharing joy and being together. It is often around a meal that we experience the happiest moments of our lives. Food is also one of the first things we turn to when life seems hard.

Women deal with food more than men do. It is something that constantly occupies their minds. Preparing food is especially important for women. Girls are taught at an early age that cooking for their family is a very important occupation, and they are praised for their skills in the kitchen. Cooking a nice meal for a man is a way of showing love. It is also most appreciated. (How many times have you heard that 'the way to a man's heart is through his stomach'?) Women are supposed to be able to cook, and do it well. A woman who does not know how to cook is considered to be lacking in femininity. As mothers, women care for their children by trying to make sure that they eat in a healthy way.

Eating is tied up with a lot of strong emotions. It is something most people turn to for comfort when they are sad, lonely, bored, disappointed or frustrated. It is like a drug. And it works! Who has not found great consolation in a slab of chocolate cake? For a moment, you forget your negative feelings and experience the pleasure of putting food that you love into your mouth. It gives you energy and is associated with relaxation and enjoyment. This would not be so bad if it only happened occasionally.

The problem is that you want to feel this pleasure nearly all the time. It has nothing to do with actual hunger. If you only wanted to satisfy hunger, it would be easy. You could simply fill up on foods that are healthy and do not make you fat. It is not eating that causes you to get fat, but *what* you eat and *why*.

Most people know what type of foods they should avoid in order not to get fat or increase their cholesterol. Even so, it seems impossible for most of us to stay away from chocolate, chips, cream, cheese, biscuits and other calorie-bombs. We simply crave them. Why? It is partly genetic. In prehistoric times, when food was scarce, human beings had a strong instinct to consume fat and sugar. These foods were rare in those days, and when they were found, had to be consumed at once to add to the human energy stores. It was important to do this for survival.

 ## Going on a binge

Most people experience moments in their lives when eating gets out of control. Indeed, many of us find it hard to stop when presented with food that we find delicious. Some people even have to give up certain things because, when presented with them, they cannot stop. (I have banned chocolate from the house for this very reason.) There are also times when we feel like eating large amounts of just about anything. We often eat just for the pleasure of tasting good food. Eating like this has nothing to do with hunger or nutrition. We use our taste buds as tools for pleasure, rather like listening to beautiful music or looking at paintings.

Sometimes we do this to relieve boredom. After all, taste is one of the five senses. (Getting pleasure from the other four, however, does not interfere with our body shape.)

There are sometimes moments in life when food is our only friend, the one consolation for stress or sadness. We eat a large amount of food, trying to get rid of the frustration. This is often followed by strong feelings of guilt. Bulimia, an eating disorder, is binge-eating carried to an extreme. It is often the cause of feelings of rejection or loss. The sufferer will eat to bursting point, and then induce vomiting. Normal bingeing, however, can be controlled with self-discipline and will-power. Understanding why we sometimes have the need to overeat may make it easier to control it.

##  Likes and dislikes

'Jack Spratt would eat no fat, his wife would eat no lean' goes the old nursery rhyme. Most people have preferences for certain foods and dislike of others. If you look at people around you at dinner parties, you will see that some people eat no vegetables, some leave the meat at the side of their plate, others cannot stand the smell of garlic or the sight of cauliflower. In England and Ireland cheese is served after the dessert, in France before; both traditions are convinced that their way is the best.

How is it possible for adults to have such different tastes? It seems that you can partly blame your parents for your eating habits. You are born with a built-in partiality for sugar and salt. New research shows that you are also born with different levels of sensitivity in your taste buds. The way you experience these two tastes is very individual. If you have a high level of sensitivity for sugar, you are satisfied with very small amounts. But if your level of sensitivity is low, you need a much larger amount of sugar to satisfy you. The same applies to salt.

These inbuilt inclinations can be altered by your parents' influence. Your love of certain foods, and the way you like to eat them, can be traced back to your childhood. It all depends on what and how your parents fed you. You may have been born with a liking for hard and crunchy things. Whether you now tend towards healthy options like raw carrots and apples, or unhealthy options like biscuits and sweets, depends on what your parents gave you to eat at an early age.

The number of times you were exposed to certain foods is also an important factor. If you were served cabbage and bacon at regular intervals as a child, chances are that you will like it as an adult, even if you turned your nose up at it the first time it was served. Research shows that the more you are exposed to a dish, the more you end up enjoying it. Most of the food and drink adults enjoy are acquired tastes. Your first gulp of beer, slug of wine, lump of blue cheese or slice of smoked salmon was probably not particularly enjoyable. These are all things you get used to little by little and learn to love because of the circumstances in which you have them.

Parents often use food as a treat. Chocolate, sweets, cakes and ice-cream are used as treats in many families. Children are even taught to comfort eat: 'Have a piece of cake to make you feel better', or 'You are a good boy, have some chocolate.' If the weather is bad, children are invited to sit in front of the fire with a biscuit or a piece of cake. Lots of adults find solace in food because of these early habits. If snacking was encouraged in your childhood home, you are much more inclined to want to eat between meals as an adult. Children who are allowed to eat in front of the television will always find pleasure in this habit.

Some foods are associated with happy times in your life. If your mother gave you a treat such as ice-cream with chocolate sauce when you felt down, you may want to relive that moment of being cared for at times when things are tough. Some people think chips taste better eaten out of a paper bag, because it reminds them of when as children they were eating such foods with their friends. Most families eat certain foods only on special occasions. They are usually full of fat and sugar, and are strongly associated with happy feelings and togetherness. When we feel sad or bored, we try to relive those happy moments. People who are busy doing something they love to do usually do not have to pig out like this. While it is unhealthy to eat too much of foods that make you fat, there is no harm in the occasional treat.

##  Food cravings

Almost all women, and about 10 per cent of men, experience cravings for certain foods as often as four times a month. This is largely due to hormonal changes in the body. Women with pre-menstrual syndrome (PMS) usually have strong cravings for chocolate and other sweet food, and also caffeine. These foods relieve tension, depression, anger and confusion. (It is safer for their environment if PMS sufferers are allowed to satisfy their cravings.) These women's consumption of certain vitamins and minerals changes during these periods. There is an increase in vitamin D, potassium, phosphorus and magnesium, and a decrease in vitamin C. Experts believe that these cravings are the body's way of demanding what it needs.

The majority of women with strong cravings report that they want to have chocolate during this time. That is probably due to the many highly stimulating ingredients that chocolate contains. Men with cravings mostly want pizza. (Why is that so hard to take seriously?) Even women who do not suffer from PMS feel more like eating sweets during the week before their period.

##  Food can change your mood

Another reason for your love of certain foods is that they can change your mood, either physiologically through changes in the brain, or psychologically by associations with your past. Chocolate, for instance, contains active compounds which affect the central nervous system. These include theobromine and phenylethamine, which has been found to relieve depression. Phenylethamine is also found in some cheeses.

Many people say they feel less depressed after a meal high in carbohydrates. Indeed, studies show that food such as pasta can reduce anger, get rid of tension

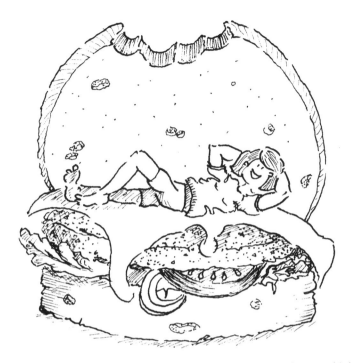

and lift fatigue. Foods with a high sugar content give you an instant kick of energy. (Sugar is pure carbohydrate.) The explanation is that carbohydrates (especially starch) increase the amount of tryptophan in the brain. Tryptophan is an amino acid that converts to serotonin, which is a chemical in the brain that controls moods. If you do not have enough serotonin in your brain, you will feel depressed, stressed, anxious, irritable, angry and even confused. People who overeat in the evening are trying to increase their serotonin levels in order to feel relaxed enough to get a good night's sleep.

Carbohydrates eaten on their own increase the level of serotonin in the brain, but if you mix them with too much protein, the process is blocked. Protein contains amino acids, other than tryptophan, which interfere with the production of serotonin. Most people who are trying to get the effect of increased serotonin do not know what foods to eat, and, as a result, choose the wrong foods. That is why they have to eat large amounts before they get the right effect. This is often the reason behind binge-eating.

#  Your eating habits

New York dietician Dr Stephen P. Gullo, author of *Thin Tastes Better*, splits eaters up into four categories: Pickers, Prowlers, Hoarders and Finishers. He maintains that if you can find your type, you can change your eating habits.

### ❭ The Picker

This person eats three meals a day and also snacks from morning to night.

How to stop snacking? Do not eat on your feet. If you eat standing, you do not pay attention to what you are eating. Eat finger foods with your left hand if you are right handed, and vice versa. This way you will think twice before you nibble.

### ❭ The Prowler

This person also snacks all day, but never eats proper meals. Eating at mealtimes is a waste of time to these people.

If you are a prowler, try to change your eating habits to more regular ones. Take time for proper meals. Make mealtimes enjoyable by laying the table with nice crockery and glasswear. Do not eat while watching television. Force yourself to pay attention to what you eat. Spend time cooking nice meals.

### ❭ The Hoarder

This type puts off eating during the day because of a lack of time and gorges at night. Hoarders tend to choose the wrong type of food because they are too hungry to pay attention to healthy choices.

If this applies to you, change your eating habits at once. Eat three meals a day, and pay special attention to breakfast. A good breakfast is the best start to the day, and it gives you energy to cope with a busy morning. Do not reward yourself for missed meals. If you are hungry, you are more likely to eat too many calories.

❯ **The Finisher**

Were you brought up to be proud of a clean plate? ('Think of all the starving children.') You sometimes even clean other people's plates.

The solution? Try to take small helpings as you will feel compelled to eat everything. Eat slowly, and allow a minimum of twenty minutes for your meal. Order something light when eating out. Do not worry about other people — let them deal with their own platefuls. (It is rude, in any case, to take food from your neighbour's plate.)

 # Think thin

Experts now believe that most people burn energy at roughly the same rate. Your metabolism starts to slow down around the age of forty. Exercise speeds it up. Apart from those two factors, let us assume that it is your eating habits, your attitude to food and your level of physical activity that are the three most important influences when it comes to body shape. The explanation for the fact that some people eat too much must lie in their eating habits and their attitude to food.

People often say about a thin woman: 'She is so lucky, she can eat what she wants without putting on an ounce.' Most thin women are, in fact, likely to be physically active, which speeds up their metabolism. Exercise keeps your metabolism high and improves the energy-burning of your muscles. Thin women may not seem to be training for the Olympics. They simply move their bodies more than fat women. They take the stairs instead of the lift. They do errands on foot rather than by car or do physical activities they enjoy that fit into their day. But the main reason they are thin is not luck or genes, but that *they have trained themselves to think about food in a way that keeps the weight off.* Thin women have a relaxed attitude to food. They do not have feelings of guilt about having a treat now and then.

Women with a weight problem often think they eat very little and are surprised that they keep putting on weight. 'I live on salad and still cannot lose weight', you often hear them complain. Overweight women have a false idea of how much they eat and what kind of food makes them fat. (Salad can be fattening if you put on too much dressing.) They also have a tendency to binge out of frustration with their weight problem. Some women even eat in secret, because they think that if nobody can see them, it will not have the same effect. This is, of course, not true. Indeed, what you eat in secret, you will have to wear in public! Chubby women often think that they are taking enough exercise by walking very slowly once a week, or buying membership to a health club and then attending classes only occasionally.

## ❱ Controlling portions

Heavy people often eat the same foods as thin people, but their portions are bigger. Thin women *do* eat things like cheese and chocolate, but in small amounts. They prefer to have a little of a high-fat food than low-fat substitutes. But the amounts are *small*. That way their craving is satisfied without piling on the weight. Most people would define a 'meal' as meaning potatoes, meat and vegetables followed by dessert. Thin people would often have just soup and an apple, or salad and cheese. You do not always need to eat a big meal just because you are sitting down to eat.

## ❱ Occasional overeating

Everybody overeats sometimes, but thin women have ways of cutting short their eating binges. One way to overcome bingeing is to do something that occupies your hands. Activities that cannot be combined with eating, such as playing the piano, sowing, knitting or painting, are good ways to distract your attention from food. The craving usually passes after about ten minutes. If you find yourself polishing off the chocolates, or having a third piece of cake, do not write off the day and keep eating. Instead of telling yourself not to eat the next day, walk for half an hour after dinner.

## ❭ Calorie awareness, treats and absence of guilt

Thin women do not, as a rule, count calories. But they know how to eat in order to stay slim. Studies show that obese people tend to underestimate calories by up to 50 per cent. If you are not sure of the calorie content of certain foods, consult the labels. It is helpful to inform yourself of the fat content of foods that have no label by reading up on nutrition in the many books on this subject. 'Think thin' when you are doing the weekly food shopping. Do not buy fattening foods in bulk. If you buy an economy-size packet of biscuits or a big bag of toffees, you will probably eat them until they are gone. If you see your favourite cake on a shelf, remind yourself that if you pass it by today, it does not mean that you will never eat it.

It is important to eat slowly, because, believe it or not, it takes twenty minutes for your brain to get the message that you are full. If you wolf down your food, you have time to eat a considerable amount before you feel that you have had enough.

Thin women allow themselves the occasional treat. Some have chips or a baked potato with sour cream and other rather fattening things once or twice a week. They know that eating sensibly 80 per cent of the time is enough to keep weight in check. This way of thinking removes the feelings of guilt about certain foods and can even curb bingeing.

## ❭ Monitoring your weight

Slim women are very aware of their weight. They usually have two numbers in their minds. One is the weight they consider ideal and the other is the weight they never let themselves exceed. Those two numbers are usually only about 2.25 kg (5 pounds) apart. Thin women notice weight gain immediately, and instinctively cut back. They monitor their weight either by weighing themselves once a week or by feeling how their clothes fit. Many overweight women have clothes in three or four sizes, so they will always have clothes to fit them perfectly, even if they gain quite a large amount of weight. Thin women rely on that too-tight feeling to remind them of the fact that it is time to cut back until they have control of their weight. Their clothes are just one size and normally fit.

##  How to stay in control

Understanding how your body works and why you want to eat certain foods at certain times should help you make your eating habits more balanced. Because, as I explained earlier, your brain craves serotonin at times, it helps to know which foods to eat to satisfy this craving. It is quite possible to give your body its full amount of what it needs without putting on weight. It is simply a matter of finding out which foods contain these chemicals.

In order to keep the right balance in your eating habits, analyse what you eat: why, how and when. Armed with this information, you can then correct your bad habits and change your diet for the better. Eating in a healthy way will seem easy and enjoyable. You will probably enjoy your food more and feel a lot better as a result. Everybody is different: needs and feelings vary from person to person. There is no universal recipe that suits everybody. It is up to each individual to find his or her particular solution.

##  Common problems and how to solve them

### ❭ Carbohydrate cravings that are hard to satisfy

People who are stressed out and grumpy towards the end of the afternoon and snack on sweets and crisps do not have a lack of self-control or something wrong with their genes. They are simply obeying a powerful signal from their serotonin-starved brains: 'Feed me more carbohydrates.'

The solution is not to stop snacking, but to find low-fat foods that increase serotonin levels. Such foods include wholewheat crackers, popcorn (with no added fat) or rice cakes. You do not need large helpings of these foods to satisfy your serotonin levels. Six crackers, half a cup of popcorn or five rice cakes is usually sufficient. Do not drink Coca-Cola or other sugary drinks with your snack. Water, either still or fizzy, is the best drink. In the evening, eat a high-carbohydrate dinner. Large quantities of potatoes or pasta will make you feel full; top up your serotonin levels and stop the temptation to snack after dinner. It will also make you feel relaxed and help you sleep.

## Chocoholics anonymous

A craving for chocolate is one of the most common problems when it comes to losing weight. Chocolate contains powerful chemicals that make you feel good. It is also addictive and tastes delicious. Most people find it nearly impossible to limit their chocolate consumption to small amounts. Chocolate is not actually bad for you, apart from the fat content, but it does make you pile on the weight.

The solution? Do have the occasional chocolate, but try to keep it to a minimum. Eat dark chocolate which has a high content of cocoa butter. It also has a high concentration of the chemicals that make you feel good. Chocolate contains vitamins and minerals such as iron and magnesium. Women have an increased need for these just before their period. Taking extra magnesium and iron in the form of vitamin supplements could help curb the need for large amounts of chocolate during this time.

## Eating out

Eating in restaurants should not cause too many problems if it occurs only occasionally. In that case, it is quite all right to indulge, forget about low fat and enjoy yourself. The next day, go back to your healthy eating habits and walk a bit further than usual. If, however, you eat out more than once a week, you have to develop a strategy to keep your fat intake low.

Always choose a low-fat starter, such as a salad with the dressing on the side or soup. For the main course, make sure you pick something without a cream sauce.

Red sauce is often based on tomato or red wine and is usually low in fat. Avoid dishes that are described as creamed, au gratin, scalloped, en casserole, pan fried, basted, braised, stewed, marinated in oil or buttery. Do not be shy about turning down hollandaise sauce, Béarnaise sauce or mayonnaise. Have a baked potato (minus the butter) instead of chips, and skip the dessert or have fruit salad.

Beware of the buffet! It is one of the worst things you can be faced with when trying to keep your weight down. Scan the whole table before you put anything on your plate. Pick things you are sure contain little fat and be careful not to end up with enough food for five people. Dishes made with mayonnaise, such as coleslaw, pasta salad or potato salad, are to be avoided.

## Shopping

You are normally presented with the maximum amount of temptation in the supermarket. The best way to deal with this is to always shop with a list. And remember, never go shopping when you are hungry. If you do, you are more likely to shop impulsively and to fill your trolley with high-fat foods you can do without. Do not buy sweets, biscuits or high-fat snacks for the children because you think they like them. If such foods are in the house, you are likely to eat them too, and the children do not need them any more than you do. Fruit is a much better snack than sweets or crisps, and the children will soon learn to like it.

## TV dinners

Never eat in front of the television. Many people who have a habit of eating while watching television overeat because they lose count of what they have eaten. They also associate television with food. This way they are unable to watch a programme without chewing on something. You should always eat at a nicely laid table. It is important to enjoy food and to eat slowly.

## Frustration with your shape can make you overeat

Many women lose patience and go back to their old unhealthy eating habits after a number of weeks on a diet. They feel frustrated when the hoped-for miracle does not happen at once. Some are disappointed because they cannot change their basic body shape. It is important to set realistic goals as you change your lifestyle and way of eating.

You are bound to fail if you feel that you must lose ten pounds in a week and promise yourself never to eat unhealthy foods. Nobody has that much discipline! *You should think of healthy eating as a long-term and permanent approach to food.* This way you will keep excess weight off for the rest of your life. You are more likely to succeed if you are honest with yourself and stick to what you can do. Your new lifestyle has to be enjoyable, not just healthy. (It is also important not to bore your friends and family by being a health fanatic!)

## Eating out of boredom

Many women overeat when they are bored or lonely. A boring afternoon seems more bearable if you eat something you like. This is usually something sweet. Carrot sticks or pieces of cucumber do not give the same pleasure. When you are bored, try to think of something to *do* rather than something to eat. Read a book or a magazine, watch television, rent a video or call a friend for a chat. Try to get out of the frame of mind that only eating gives comfort. It is something that you learned in early childhood which you have to wean yourself off.

## Have a treat once a week

This was something that worked for me when I had to lose a lot of weight: taking one day a week off healthy food. I allowed myself all the things I should not eat and that I longed for on that day. I had chocolate, chips, cream and other forbidden foods. The rest of the time, I stuck seriously to a low-fat diet. This way, it was easier to stay away from fattening foods, since I knew that I could have them once a week.

I had something to look forward to and did not feel deprived. I still follow this rule and my weight has stayed the same ever since.

##  How to succeed without pain

~ Remember that you *can* do it.
~ Make sure you are physically active every day.
~ Set realistic goals.
~ Take it one day at a time.
~ Eat three meals a day and allow yourself a (fat-free) snack in the afternoon.
~ Find out which foods are satisfying and filling without making you put on weight.
~ Have one diet-free day a week.
~ Eat slowly.
~ Be aware of fat in your food.
~ Nip weight gain in the bud. Take off the pounds before they become a permanent fixture.
~ Do not keep junk food in the house.
~ Always shop with a list and when you are not hungry.
~ Never eat in front of the television.
~ Do not 'reward' yourself with high-fat foods after exercising.
~ Eat at least five helpings of fruit and vegetables a day.
~ Do not buy fattening food in bulk.
~ Redefine the word 'meal'.
~ Throw out your big-size clothes.

If you follow these rules, it will not be long before your friends say: 'You are so lucky to be naturally thin!'

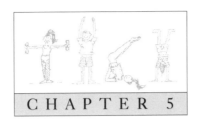

## CHAPTER 5

# WORKING OUT IS HARD TO DO

The most important thing you can do for good health is to be physically active. Inactivity is an even greater threat to your health than smoking. A physically active smoker has better health than an inactive non-smoker. (Imagine the state of health of an inactive smoker!) Most people are aware of the benefits of exercise. Sadly, the resistance to physical activity is a very common problem. While it is true that the human body was designed to move, it also has a strong instinct to remain immobile. This instinct was important in prehistoric times, because food was scarce and humans had to conserve energy in order to survive. These days, your food intake is constant. You need to work your body and use up stored energy.

Modern life has forced us to adopt a largely inactive life, and we have to make an effort to find the time and energy to be physically active. It is astonishing how inventive most people are when it comes to finding excuses for not taking exercise. Most people find it cruel to keep battery hens in a state of total immobility. But they are doing exactly the same to their own bodies. If people in general knew how bad it is to neglect the body's need for exercise, they would not be so ready to flop on the sofa after a day at the office.

You often hear that you should ask your doctor before starting an exercise programme. This is an outdated notion that keeps many people from pursuing an activity that would boost their health. Exercise is much safer than inactivity in terms of health and well-being. Rather than seeking permission to exercise, you should have to get permission to be sedentary, because inactivity is far more dangerous. Even at an advanced age, if you are generally well, it is not necessary to seek your doctor's approval for moderate activities such as walking, gentle muscle toning or doubles tennis. (You should see your doctor if you have undiagnosed symptoms such as fainting spells or shortness of breath, or other signs that there may be something seriously wrong.) While sedentary people who decide to run a marathon need to check with their doctor, you do not need to consult one to go out and take a walk.

##  Common excuses for not taking exercise

### 〉 'I do not have the time to exercise.'

This is the most common excuse of all. Well, you have to make the time, because exercise is one of the most important ingredients in a healthy lifestyle. If you never take any exercise at all, you will soon develop health problems. These problems may not appear serious at first, but they will get worse with time. As most people manage to do what they want in their free time, such as going to the cinema, watching television, having a drink in the pub or going out for a meal, it should not be difficult to fit in a little physical activity. You also waste time doing unnecessary things every day, for example talking nonsense on the telephone or watching mindless junk on television. With a little planning, you should be able to fit in some physical activity each day.

### 〉 'Exercise is boring.'

I hear this excuse nearly as often as the previous one. All exercise is not boring. It is just a matter of finding something that you enjoy. You do not have to jog or swim if you do not like it. There are many sports that are very enjoyable. Some people like sports that require skill, such as tennis or golf. Others do not want to have to think about what they are doing.In that case, try walking. Some hobbies involve a lot of physical effort, but they are not considered to be a sport. Dancing, be it tap, ballroom or disco dancing, is an excellent way to keep active. There are so many activities that are easily available these days.

### 'Exercise does not make you thin, so what is the point?'

Being fit is not about being thin. It is wrong to exercise just to be thin. Fitness is important for your health. Thin people often think that they do not have to exercise. This is false. It is not the size of your thighs or your waist measurement that decides your need for physical activity. Indeed, a fat, active person is healthier than someone who is thin and inactive. Thin or fat, you need to work your heart, lungs and circulation, and put all the muscles and joints through their full range of motion in order to remain healthy.

### 'Exercise hurts.'

While you have to expect some stiffness and pain at the beginning of an exercise programme, if you have previously been totally inactive, there is no discomfort at all when you get used to an active lifestyle. You should never continue an exercise that hurts while you are doing it. The saying 'no pain, no gain', so common in the 1970s, is totally wrong. If it hurts, do not do it. In any case, it is not necessary to work out to the limit of your endurance in order to be basically fit. Moderate exercise, provided it is done regularly, is just as beneficial.

### 'I was good at sports in my youth, so I must still have some fitness left.'

Fitness and muscle strength cannot be stored. You cannot be fit if you do not exercise regularly now, irrespective of what you did in school. Although the skills related to some sports, such as swimming and cycling, will always remain, the fitness associated with any activity is lost within three weeks of giving it up. A good swimmer or cyclist will be stiff and sore when taking up the sport again after an absence of only a few weeks. Continuity is the key to a good level of fitness.

### ❭ 'I am too tired and I have a headache.'

If you feel tired after work, exercise will give you more energy than that which you imagine you gain by just sitting on the sofa after dinner. A fit person has twice the energy of an inactive one. When you are inactive, your blood circulation slows down, and there is less oxygen in your blood. Your inactive muscles cannot convert carbohydrate into energy. That is why you feel tired. A headache is often caused by bad circulation, and an activity such as walking may relieve it. Indeed, if you take regular exercise, you will have fewer headaches. Many women do not want to exercise during their period. Doing something active during this time has been proven to relieve a lot of discomfort: it can even stop stomach cramps. You should never exercise, however, when you are ill.

### ❭ 'I am too old.'

It is never too late to start exercising. The older you are, the more you need to keep active. It is possible for people even in their eighties and nineties to improve stamina and muscle strength. In a recent study in Sweden, a group of people aged between eighty-five and ninety-five who trained with weights for eight weeks improved their muscle strength by an average of 30 per cent.

Older people tend to become more and more passive. The reason for the famous 'middle-age spread' is merely decreasing activity and increasing fat-intake at an age when your metabolism slows down. What a recipe for disaster! Many people look forward to their old age as a time when they no longer have to do anything physically active. This is seen as normal and acceptable. The opposite should be the case. Old people should take exercise every day. It is the only way to escape many of the uncomfortable symptoms of ageing.

# What regular exercise does for you

It:

~ Reduces the risk of heart disease by improving blood circulation throughout the body

~ Keeps weight under control

~ Improves blood cholesterol levels

~ Prevents and manages high blood pressure

~ Prevents bone loss

~ Boosts energy levels

~ Helps manage stress

~ Releases tension

~ Improves the ability to fall asleep quickly and sleep well

~ Improves self-image

~ Counters anxiety and depression, and increases enthusiasm and optimism

~ Increases muscle strength, giving greater capacity for other physical activities

~ Helps delay or prevent chronic illnesses and diseases associated with ageing in older people, and maintains quality of life and independence longer

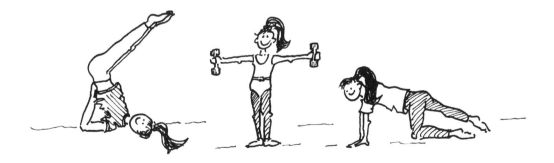

# Myths and truths about exercise

| Myth | Truth |
| --- | --- |
| Exercise makes you lose weight. | Exercise makes you lose inches and fat. But as muscles weigh more than fat, the weighing scales may not reflect the lost fat. (You may even get heavier.) |
| Exercise makes you eat less. | Exercise stimulates your appetite. You must pay attention to what you eat at all times. |
| Hard work will soon show results. | You will see results, but it may take longer than you think. It can take up to a month before you notice an improvement. Patience is important. |
| You must sweat and suffer to get fit. | Moderate exercise makes you fit, provided it is done regularly. |
| A supple person is fit. | A supple person is just supple. Fitness can only be achieved with regular exercise. |
| Thin people do not need exercise. | Everybody needs exercise! |
| If you exercise, you can eat what you like. | Unless you are training for a marathon, you still have to cut down on fat. Exercise has to be combined with a low-fat diet for good health and weight management. |

 # How to fit fitness in

As a supposed lack of time seems to be the most common obstacle for people when it comes to taking regular exercise, fitting physical activity into your daily life is the best solution. It is not true that working out in a gym and going to an aerobics class are the only activities that count as exercise. The idea is to put more physical effort into your day. Anything that makes your heart beat a little faster and makes you work your muscles is exercise. Whether you are a housewife working at home or a career woman with a long day at the office, it is possible to get in quite a lot of exercise if you reorganise your routine a little.

## At home, you should:

~ Do housework yourself instead of hiring a cleaning lady

~ Work in the garden or mow the grass; using a riding mower does not count!

~ Rake leaves, dig and prune

~ Go out for a short walk before dinner or breakfast or both! (Start with five to ten minutes and increase it to thirty minutes.)

~ Walk or cycle to the corner shop

~ When watching television, sit up straight instead of lying on the sofa

~ Not use the television remote control; get up each time you want to change the channel

~ Not ask others to fetch things for you; get them yourself

~ Stand up while talking on the telephone

~ Park further away from the supermarket or shopping centre. (Carrying bags is good for your muscles.)

~ Play with your children; join in their games of football or catch

~ Put on some music and disco-dance for twenty minutes or more; the children will love it

~ Not have the television switched on all the time; consult the television guide and choose the programmes that really interest you

## At the office, you should:

~ Discuss work while taking a walk, instead of having meetings in the office

~ Walk down the hall to speak to someone instead of using the phone

~ Take the stairs instead of using the lift, or get off a few floors early and take the stairs the remainder of the way

~ Walk to the office and home — all the way, or at least part of the way

~ Walk during your lunch-hour

~ When travelling, walk while waiting for the plane

~ Stay at hotels with fitness centres or a swimming pool

~ Join a fitness centre near your office; you could work out before or after work to avoid rush-hour traffic

~ Schedule your exercise time on your business calendar and treat it as any other important appointment

**At play you should:**

~ Plan family outings and holidays that include physical activity (swimming, walking, tennis)

~ See the sights in foreign cities by walking

~ Do physical activities with friends; make this a regular occurrence

~ Dance with someone or by yourself — or take dancing lessons

~ Join a club that emphasises physical activity

~ At the beach, get up and walk rather than lying down; play beach-ball games with the children. You have no children? Borrow some!

~ Never use a cart when playing golf

~ Put up a badminton net in the garden and invite your friends to play

There are many other ways of making your life more physically active. Try to think of some yourself. Get your family and friends involved in your new lifestyle. You will do them a favour and, at the same time, have someone to push you to continue. Once you get used to being active, you will not want to stop. The feeling of well-being that exercise gives you is very addictive. Try to keep it up for a month and I guarantee that by then exercise will feel like an indispensable part of your life.

Do not overdo it. Exercise at a low to moderate level at first. You can slowly increase the duration and intensity of your activities as you become more fit. Increase the pace as you walk, and go a bit further each time. Take your time to get used to other sports. Improve your technique before you speed up. Exercise should not be exhausting, but invigorating and enjoyable.

# Walking, the best exercise for every body

Indoors or outdoors, on roads and paths, walking is the easiest and most convenient way to get fit. It is low impact and does not jar your joints or back. Walking does not require equipment, experience or membership fees. It can be done alone or with family and friends at any time and anywhere.

If you walk for thirty minutes a day, you will notice many benefits within two or three weeks, such as a sense of well-being and good mood, and an improved ability to meet the demands of a busy day. There will also be an improvement in your mobility, vitality and energy. The muscles in your shins, calves, thighs and buttocks will be firmer.

In the long term, walking every day can help you lose weight and reduce your risk of coronary heart disease. Walking increases and maintains bone density. The steady, low impact of such a weight-bearing exercise is the action that stimulates the mineral content to remain within the bone structure.

Walking just thirty minutes a day leads to a steady shedding of about 8 kg (about 18 pounds) a year. If combined with a low-fat diet and other ways of keeping physically active, the weight-loss will be considerably more. (If you take no exercise at all, your weight will increase by the same amount each year.)

### How hard should you be working?

You should train at 55 to 85 per cent of your maximum heart rate. (Your maximum heart rate is 220 minus your age.) In practice, this means a vigorous 5 to 6 km (3 to 4 miles) an hour, which allows you to carry on a conversation without getting tired or short of breath. If you walk faster, you get into oxygen debt (as explained in Chapter 2). A leisurely stroll while window-shopping or walking around the garden with a drink in your hand does not count as exercise.

Your workout intensity should be geared to your present fitness capacity. Walk slowly at first and pick up the pace as you become fitter. Avoid hills in the beginning.

After a few months, they can be an extra challenge. Always start by walking slowly the first five minutes. This allows your heart rate and blood pressure to climb gradually to your training level. At all times your walk should end with a leisurely stroll for two or three minutes to allow your cardiovascular system to get back to its pre-exercise level.

## Comfortable shoes

It is a good idea to invest in a pair of comfortable shoes. Even if your walking takes place on the way to the office, wear comfortable shoes and change into something more fashionable when you get there.

Select a lightweight walking shoe. Look for shock absorption in the heel and ball of the shoe. (Shock absorption is important to avoid heel pain and burning or tenderness in the ball of the foot.) Make sure that you choose a shoe adapted to your specific needs. If you intend to walk in rough terrain, get a walking boot that supports your ankle as well. There are many different walking shoes available in sports shops. The staff should be able to advise you on the correct footwear for you. Good shoes are an investment that you will never regret.

## A healthy environment

If the weather is warm (25°C or more), wear light clothes and modify your speed. If it is cold, dress warmly and in layers. It is best, in built-up areas, to walk early in the morning or at night to avoid air pollution. If you suffer from asthma or some other respiratory condition, check with your doctor to see how much exercise you should take. Avoid unfamiliar or potentially dangerous places. Walk on pavements or safe paths, preferably with a friend. Be careful of traffic.

## A good posture

Keep your back straight and your shoulders relaxed as you walk. Keep your chin parallel to your spine and your eyes on the horizon. Your arms should swing naturally at your sides. Maintain a natural stride and walk with a rolling, heel-to-toe foot action.

#  Streeeeeetching!

It is important to stretch out your Achilles' tendons, calves, hamstrings and quadriceps (the front of your thighs). Your back will also benefit from a good stretch. It stops you getting sore and stiff and makes you more flexible, especially at the beginning.

### Calf

Lean forward with your hands on a support (a tree or bench), arms straight. Put one foot in front of the other (your feet should be parallel and about half a metre (a foot and a half) apart, and bend the knee of the leg that is in front. Push the heel of the back leg which is straight hard into the ground and hold the stretch for thirty seconds. Then change legs and repeat the stretch.

### Achilles' tendon

Do the same thing as for the calf but bend the knee of the back leg as well, and hold.

### Hamstring

Let go of the support, straighten your back leg again and lean forward with your hands on your front thigh, just above the knee. Hold the stretch for thirty seconds and then change legs.

### Front of the thigh

Stand up straight and hold on to something with one hand for support. Bend your knee back and try to get your heel to your bottom. Pull your foot with one hand and hold, bringing your hip forward. Then change legs.

## ❭ Back

Bend forward, knees bent and back round. Grab the back of your knees with your hands and pull up, with your back still in the rounded position. Hold and repeat. (Never force a stretch. It should feel comfortable.)

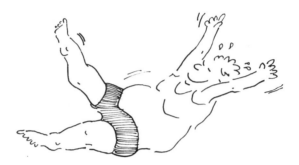

If you do no exercise at all, you are just like a battery hen. But whereas the hen is forced into total inactivity, you have a choice. Either you can stay inactive and feel your body deteriorate little by little or you can take action and gradually improve your health. If you do nothing else, try at least to walk. Although a complete fitness programme consists of aerobic activities (such as walking, running or cycling) combined with strengthening exercises for the entire body, walking alone will keep you in reasonable shape.

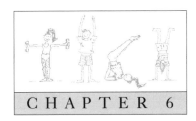

## CHAPTER 6

# FROM FLAB TO FAB

A trim figure with a slim waist, a flat stomach, the bust in the right place, thighs with good muscle-tone and well-shaped hips and bottom: that is what most women want, but very few know how to achieve it, and fewer still are prepared to do the work required.

As you age, your skin and muscles lose their elasticity and parts of the body begin to sag. If you do not make your muscles firm, the sagging gets gradually worse. Everything travels 'south': your bust tries to join your waist, your stomach hangs over the waistline of your skirts or trousers and your bottom is suddenly much lower down than it used to be. Fortunately, there *is* a solution. You can avoid the droopy look and keep a youthful figure *if you work your muscles*.

Regular exercise that tones your muscles is important for good health. If you are aerobically fit, you have energy, stamina and good circulation. But that is only half the picture. You also need to make your muscles strong and your joints supple. If you work your muscles regularly, you will improve your flexibility, mobility, coordination, balance and strength. You will have good muscle-tone.

 ## What is muscle-tone?

The World Health Organisation defines muscle-tone as 'the state of tension in a muscle when it is at *rest*'. It is no good flexing your muscles to feel their state of tension, because even an untrained muscle feels strong when tensed. Feel the muscles of your relaxed thighs. Are they hard and strong? No? It is time you did some exercise!

Muscles need to work regularly to develop and maintain strength. If you do not put your body through some kind of movement, your muscles will start to shrink. A person who has complete bed rest loses 50 per cent of muscle mass *in only eight days*. When I recently had to stay in bed with a broken leg, I saw my injured leg shrink dramatically during ten days of complete immobility. It took months to restore the muscles.

Doctors now recommend that even badly injured patients do some kind of exercise. My doctor told me to swim, and even use a rowing machine, only weeks after the accident. (I did not, however, have a cast on my leg, as a more modern form of surgery — insertion of a pin — had been used). Patients with back problems are now advised to try to exercise even if it causes some pain. (If you have severe pain, however, you must still rest until the pain eases.) The best way to prevent back and joint problems is to exercise.

## Working your muscles improves your looks

Even if you do not need, or want, to lose weight, good muscle-tone greatly improves the shape of your body. With just a little regular work, you will tone your arms, bust, waist, stomach, thighs and buttocks. You will lose inches all over and make your back straighter. Working your muscles will also improve your blood circulation and speed up your metabolism.

Toned muscles burn fat more efficiently than slack ones. A person with strong muscles burns fat efficiently, even at rest. As you get fitter and your muscles get stronger, your ability to burn fat will steadily increase.

The weighing scale is not a good indication of fat loss, as muscles weigh more than fat. You may not lose very much weight while you are getting stronger and fitter (even if you cut down drastically on fat in your diet), but you will lose inches. You will notice that your clothes start getting looser and that you look slimmer and fitter.

##  Flexibility, coordination and mobility

*Flexibility* is another word for suppleness. It is important to keep joints and muscles supple right through life in order to avoid stiffness and pain as you grow older. Some people are naturally supple, or 'double jointed'. A person's suppleness varies from 'rather stiff' to 'very supple'. If you are stiff, you can improve your suppleness with exercise. It is especially important for a person with poor flexibility to try to improve their suppleness.

*Coordination* is the ability to coordinate the different parts of your body. When you exercise, you improve the communication between nerves and muscles and you learn to use the correct group of muscles at the right moment. You also learn to move efficiently without using too much energy, and your reflexes become faster. What you learn by working your muscles in a fitness programme is useful in your daily life and other sports. For example, you learn to avoid back injuries by lowering your shoulders, bending your knees and placing your feet correctly. Good coordination is useful in all sports. It can drastically improve your performance at work as well.

Many people have reduced *mobility* in their joints and ligaments. That makes their movements stiff and slow. They get pain and discomfort in their necks, shoulders, hips and backs. Improved mobility in muscles and ligaments, which you get by exercising, increases performance and helps avoid injuries. Exercise helps 'oil the machinery' of your body. The more physically active you are, the more you will increase the flow of blood to your joints. The goal of a fitness programme is to restore the natural mobility you had when you were young.

A flat stomach

Muscles need regular exercise. You need to work them a minimum of three times a week: less than that, and you will never see an improvement. Your stomach muscles (that is, the abdominals) and back muscles are the ones that most need toning because they do not get a lot of work in the average person's daily life. Your arms get a certain amount of exercise when you do your daily chores, and if you walk and do sports regularly, your legs will get stronger. But there are few occupations (apart from ballet or gymnastics) that work the stomach muscles regularly. There is nothing more unattractive than a protruding stomach (except when you are pregnant — then it is beautiful). When your stomach muscles are slack, you look unfit and fat.

It is also important to keep these muscles strong, as they support your back. Weak abdominal muscles are a major factor in lower back pain. You need to spend only five minutes a day doing a few easy movements to get your stomach looking flatter and your muscles stronger. The toning programme at the end of this book will do just that. If you do it a minimum of three times a week, you will notice an improvement after about a month. If you keep it up, you will always have a trim waist, a flat stomach and a strong back.

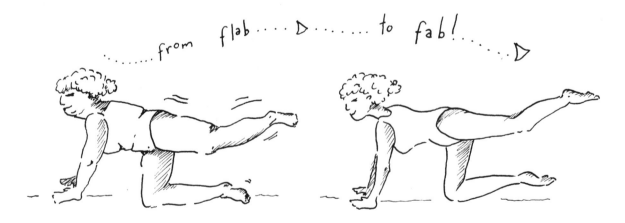
.......from flab ....▷....... to fab!.......▷

Stomach exercises will only trim the muscles in the stomach. In order to lose fat, you have to change your eating habits. Unless you cut down on fat in your food, and engage in aerobic and fat-burning activities (like walking), abdominal exercises will only trim your waistline to a certain extent. It is nearly impossible for most mature women, especially those who have given birth, to get a completely flat stomach. Abdominal exercise improves the stomach and helps you hold it in, but it will never be totally flat (unless you are exceptionally thin). A *slightly* rounded stomach is, in any case, feminine and adds to the soft charm of a woman's body.

##  The pelvic floor

The muscles which support the organs in the lower abdomen (the womb and the bladder) can often become weak after childbirth. Women are advised to exercise these muscles daily. Failure to keep these muscles firm can cause stress incontinence (urine escapes on coughing, laughing, running or jumping) and more seriously, a prolapsed womb (the womb is in a lower position than it should be). Women who are fit and take part in sports normally have strong pelvic muscles, even after several babies. New mothers are taught how to exercise the pelvic floor muscles by a midwife or physiotherapist before leaving hospital, but many forget to do so once they get home. Imagine that you have a walnut in your vagina and try to pull it up higher and hold for a moment. This is a very good exercise which should, ideally, be done at least twenty times a day if you do not exercise in any other way. If you take part in fitness classes, you would normally do exercises that tighten the pelvic floor automatically. There are exercises for your buttocks in the exercise programme at the end of the book that can be done in addition to tightening internally in the same way. If you keep the pelvic floor muscles tight, you will avoid problems in later life.

#  How to work your muscles

There are many different ways to work your muscles, such as stretching, yoga, callanetics and body-building. You will find an abundance of videos on the market for exercising at home. Then there are the 'contraptions' widely advertised on the shopping television channels.

### Stretching and yoga

Stretching and yoga are both based on the same principle: stretching out, holding the position for some time, releasing and repeating the movement. This method makes you strong and supple, without straining. It is difficult at the beginning, and some of the movements are hard, but you work within your own capacity and gradually improve your ability. Both consist of exercises that are particularly beneficial for people who suffer from stress, tension or insomnia. Women who do stretching or yoga look wonderful and age well. Try it and you will not want to stop. (By the way, you should always include some stretching in any fitness programme or sport. It prevents muscle soreness, especially when you are a beginner.)

### Callanetics

Callanetics is a method of exercising based on many repetitions of each movement. It was invented in the 1980s by a woman in America called Pinckney Callan (hence the name). The movements do not differ much from any other muscle-toning programme, but the many repetitions make it more efficient. Callanetics classes are excellent for toning muscles.

### Body-building

Body-building is probably the most efficient method for making your muscles strong and firm. Women started working out with weights and going to gyms in the 1980s and there are probably as many women as men in the gyms nowadays. Working out with weights and machines is an excellent way to tone your body. It is the best method if you want long, lean muscles all over. Body-building gives the fastest results of all muscle-toning methods. If you stick at it, you will soon have well-defined muscles.

It is important at the beginning to do the exercises with an instructor. If you are not familiar with the machines, you may injure yourself. You must also learn the correct way to place your body for the various exercises. Once you know how to work out on the various machines, you can do it on your own. The advantage with this way of exercising is that you can go when it suits you and you do not have to be on time for a specific class. However, many women start going to the gym with the best of intentions, but give up after only a few sessions (I am one of them). The exercises are very hard, and many gyms are so crowded that you have to queue for each machine. You need a lot of self-discipline to follow a body-building programme regularly.

Some women are worried that working out with machines will give them big, bulging muscles. It won't. Female body-builders with big muscles have to take steroids, in addition to working out for two to three hours a day, in order to develop big muscles.

### Exercise videos

Exercise videos can be found in bookshops and larger newsagents. Most of them are good, but you have to know what to look for. Aerobic videos are a good choice if you cannot get out to walk regularly. The most common problem with them, however, is that they usually give you an aerobic workout, with only a few minutes for toning muscles at the end. It is best to look for an all-over toning programme, like Callanetics. If you combine this with regular walking, your fitness routine is complete. Unfortunately, most of the videos are quite long, taking about forty-five minutes on average. If you are too busy to go to classes, you may not have time to follow a video that takes this amount of time to complete. Try to find one that takes about twenty minutes.

Avoid videos made by actresses, supermodels and other celebrities. They normally have no knowledge of fitness, and, although lovely to watch, some are positively dangerous.

### ❩ That 'thing' under your bed

There are many 'contraptions' for toning your muscles on the market, usually advertised on television. There is the 'ab coach', which consists of a metal frame that helps you work your stomach muscles. 'The bun and thigh toner' is also made of metal with springs to give you resistance as you work the muscles on your thighs and buttocks. The advertisements tell you to work your 'abs', your 'buns' or your 'butt'. You may think that new parts of the body have been invented. Do not worry, these are only American expressions for your good old stomach, thighs and bottom.

There are many more gadgets with equally inventive names to lure you to part with your money. They all 'store easily under your bed'. Most are probably very good, and would give excellent results. However, exercise experts in America have found that these devices are no more efficient than exercising *without* equipment. The only benefit lies in their motivation value. Someone who has paid up to £200 for a metal gadget is more likely to exercise regularly. However, if you are a couch potato with great resistance to exercise, you are not likely to use a machine like this for long (even if it is lurking under your bed). Studies show that the average buyer uses any of these machines no more than seven times. In any case, you must have a different apparatus for each part of the body. For a total workout, you would need a minimum of three different machines.

##  Other ways of toning muscles

Many sports and hobbies tone your muscles. Some give you an all-over muscle-tone, while others tone the muscles on specific parts of the body.

## Upper body

At a time when fitness professionals are constantly talking about the advantages of regular, moderate exercise, *gardening* is being recognised as a healthy hobby that can provide significant benefits to people of all ages. Depending on the activity, gardening can be as strenuous as lifting weights. Tasks such as digging, raking and planting are equivalent to brisk walking. Mowing the lawn with a push mower, chopping wood and tilling are as difficult as hill walking or playing doubles tennis. Gardeners also have the advantage that, usually enjoying their activity, they do not think of it as exercise.

*Housework* may not be as much fun as gardening (and it could not possibly be described as a hobby), but it does make you physically active. Chores like making beds, hoovering and washing floors and windows have to be done on a regular basis. These jobs will give you lots of opportunities to work the muscles in your arms and shoulders. DIY jobs like painting and putting up wallpaper have the same effect — and think of the money you will save by not paying someone else to do it.

## Legs, buttocks and thighs

Cycling, walking and jogging work your lower body. They give good muscle-tone and also burn fat efficiently.

*Cycling* gives you firm muscles in your thighs, calves and buttocks. It is an aerobic exercise that is not weight-bearing. It gives you a good level of cardiovascular fitness (heart, lungs and circulation). Moreover, it is a great way to get around a crowded town or city. You save a lot of time by avoiding traffic jams and looking for a parking space. And it is also good for the environment.

*Walking and jogging* are more complete forms of exercise because they are also weight-bearing. Walking is probably better than jogging, because you get to the fat stores in your body immediately (as I explained in Chapter 2). Your thighs and bottom become firm when you walk regularly. It is also more convenient to fit walking into your day, in contrast to more organised sports such as jogging, where you have to spend time showering and changing your clothes. Jogging is nevertheless a very good way of keeping fit. If you run for half an hour three to four times a week you will have a good level of fitness. However, as with other vigorous sports, jogging makes you sweat; some people find this unpleasant, and many women do not like to mess up their hair.

It is important to know that although walking is a less demanding sport than jogging, it makes you nearly as fit. Many people believe that running is the only way to fitness, and, as they do not want to jog, do nothing.

### ❭ All-over muscle-tone

*Swimming* is an excellent sport which combines all-over muscle-tone with aerobic exercise. If you swim three times a week, you will be very fit indeed. It is not a weight-bearing exercise, however, which you need to take into account for your complete health picture. (Swim for twenty minutes three times a week and do the same amount of walking, and you have a total fitness routine.) The problem with swimming is, again, time. You have to go to the pool, change, get wet, shower and change again. And what about your hair?

*Rowing machines* are excellent, and the only machine that gives you an all-over workout for your muscles, heart and lungs. However, it is not a weight-bearing exercise, and so you should still walk regularly to keep your bones strong.

*Horse riding* is not weight-bearing either, but makes you fit in all other respects. It gives you great muscle-tone (especially in your legs, thighs, buttocks, shoulders and arms) plus aerobic fitness. If you are experienced, riding three times a week or more, you will be very fit indeed.

*Badminton, tennis and cross-country skiing* are all weight-bearing and as near to a complete exercise routine for the whole body as you will get. You may have to add a few abdominal exercises to keep your waist and stomach slim and trim. Sadly, few people (except Scandinavians) have access to regular cross-country skiing. Fortunately, you can play badminton and tennis well into old age, changing to doubles games as you grow older.

*Golf* is also a weight-bearing exercise, but it is the walking, not hitting the ball, that is beneficial in this case.

##  The busy woman's toning programme

The toning programme you will find at the end of this book is the *minimum* you need to do for basic muscle-tone. If you do it at least three times a week (or ideally, every second day), your muscles will get stronger and firmer. The exercises will trim your waist, flatten your stomach and tone your bust, thighs and buttocks. At the end of the programme, you stretch out the muscles you have used, to improve flexibility and reduce soreness. (I deliberately do not include exercises for the arms, because I believe that they get a certain amount of work in your daily activities. I am aiming for the shortest possible workout.)

It is a good idea to do the exercises first thing in the morning. It is a wonderful way to start the day. It improves your circulation and gives you energy for the day ahead.

You will burn only a few calories (mostly from the carbohydrate stores in your muscles) while you are working out, but as your muscles get stronger, their ability to burn fat will improve. I use this way of keeping my muscles in trim when I am on holiday or cannot do my normal classes for other reasons. Once you learn the programme by heart, you will always be able to work your muscles wherever you are. You can do the exercises in your living-room or bedroom, in a hotel room, at the beach or in the garden. The full programme takes fifteen minutes.

Start slowly, with just a few repetitions of each exercise. Increase the intensity as you get stronger. When the whole programme seems easy to do, increase the number of repetitions. In time, it will seem so easy and natural that you may even want to do it *every day*! It will be a month to six weeks before you see any improvement, but you will *feel* much stronger after only three weeks.

I have given this programme to many of my friends, who have been delighted with the results. If you previously did not work your muscles, the effect will be spectacular!

##  The ouch! factor

Most people have experienced soreness in their muscles after unaccustomed exercise or strenuous activity. You may have started gardening with great enthusiasm on a spring day after a winter of relative inactivity. Or someone suggested a game of tennis and you may not have played for a long time. If you take to the ski slopes without preparing your muscles with some exercise, or go riding after a long absence, the result is the same. This painful feeling is caused by tiny tears in the muscles, which heal quickly with care. If this happens to you, rest the next day, and go back to gentle exercise for a few sessions before you increase the intensity. If you return to total inactivity, the result will only be even stiffer muscles.

When you start an activity or sport you are not used to, it is important that you do it slowly and gently at the beginning. If you ease yourself into an activity, you will not be sore or stiff. Try to exercise every second day to give your muscles a chance to recover between sessions. You will feel the effect of the exercise in your muscles, but without pain. You should also warm up for a few minutes before doing any type of exercise, and finish with some gentle stretching. This way you prepare the muscles for the work to come, and cool them down slowly at the end.

In an exercise class, work at your own pace. This means that you only do as many repetitions as you can manage comfortably. It is quite all right to do a few repetitions, rest for a minute, and continue for another few. Do not try to keep up with the person standing next to you, who may have been going to the class for years. It is a class, not a competition! The same applies to stretching. There are some women who look as if they are made of rubber and can tie themselves in knots. Do not try to do the same. Many fitness teachers make the mistake of stretching their bodies to the extreme (some like to show off in this way). It is hard for the majority of people to follow their example. A stretch should feel comfortable and *never* hurt.

You should not let others push you into working harder or faster than you are comfortable with in any sport or activity; this could even lead to accidents in some cases. In sports where safety depends on your ability and strength, such as horse riding, swimming and downhill skiing, you should always work within *your own* limits. Some people love to compete. Do not be tempted to join in.

If you get a cramp, which usually occurs in your legs or feet, walk around until the pain eases. A cramp is a spasm in a muscle that is worked too hard. It usually happens when you start a sport or activity that you are not used to.

##  Staying in shape

If you work your muscles regularly, you will always look well. You can stay trim and fit well into old age. I know women in their seventies and eighties who look and feel wonderful because they are physically active. Whatever your weight or shape, firm muscles are better than slack ones. If you pick an activity that you enjoy, it will not seem difficult to achieve good muscle-tone. Try different activities, even some you have never tried before, in order to find something that suits you. Who knows, you may even get hooked on exercise! If you have never experienced the feeling of stretching and working all the muscles in your body, you will be surprised what a pleasure it is.

You do not have to do the same activity all the time. It is just as beneficial to do different exercises each time. You could do yoga on Mondays, swim on Wednesdays and do Callanetics on Fridays. As long as you work all your muscles each time, three times a week, it does not matter what you choose.

Muscles lose their strength very quickly. If you have to stop exercising for a while, make sure that you are not inactive for too long. Ballerinas say: 'Miss a day's training and you can feel it, miss two and your teacher can see it, miss three and the audience can see it.' If you are not a ballerina, a week off will not make a lot of difference. Once you have attained a good level of fitness, it is fairly easy to maintain it, even with an occasional break of a week. If you have been away from exercise for over two weeks, however, you must resume your normal programme gradually.

**For good muscle tone you should:**
~ Work out at least three times a week
~ Choose something you enjoy
~ Start slowly, and increase the pace as you get fitter
~ Warm up at the beginning and stretch at the end of any sport or activity
~ Do the exercises correctly, keeping your back straight
~ Never do anything that hurts. (Exercise should be an effort, but should never hurt.)
~ Never exercise when you are ill
~ Make sure you do not stop for more than a week
~ Go back gradually if you have not been exercising for more than two weeks
~ Do the programme shown at the end of the book, if you have little time for anything else

Muscles are like rubber bands. They can have poor elasticity with no strength to keep anything up, or they can be strong and tight. When the force of gravity pulls parts of your body down, a little exercise will help prevent this, and, in fact, make a great difference. If you want your bust and your bottom to stay where they were when you were younger, exercise is the only way. To get from flab to fab takes a certain amount of time and effort, but it is well worth it!

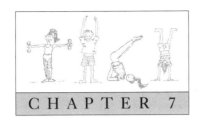

## CHAPTER 7

# BACK AGAIN!

The main cause of back problem is that we walk on our hind legs, instead of on all fours as we were designed to do. The spine is fragile and not really suited to this. But the upright position that the human race adopted many thousands of years ago should not damage your back, provided your muscles are strong enough to support it.

Eight out of ten adults experience back pain at some time during their lives. It is a recurring problem for many. Back pain can make your life miserable and prevent you from working, sleeping and doing things that you enjoy. It is the main cause of absenteeism in the workforce in most countries. As it is impossible to go back to walking on all fours, adopting the right habits is the only solution. Most people do not know what those are, and that is the main cause of pain and stiffness in the back.

In this chapter I will look at common problems and what to do about them. It *is* possible to have a problem-free back. If you take some exercise, correct your bad habits and learn how to stand, sit and lie correctly, you can look forward to a pain-free and enjoyable life. (I have myself had serious backache, but since I learned how to align my body correctly and eliminate some bad habits, my back has been in good condition.)

## The basic structure

Your spine consists of twenty-four vertebrae plus your coccyx, which has a few additional vertebrae that are fused together. There are discs made out of soft cartilage between each vertebra. These discs, which act as shock absorbers, become more brittle and fragile with age or inactivity.

There is a hole in the centre of each disc for the bone marrow. There are, in addition, spaces between the vertebrae for the nerves that connect to different parts of the body. The discs have no blood supply, which makes them a weak link in the musculoskeletal system. Physical activity is therefore important in order to keep the discs supple. (When you move about, you improve the nutrition to the cells in the discs.)

There are a number of muscles attached to the spine. Their purpose is to support it and keep it in the right position. There are, in addition, strong ligaments which also help support and stabilise your back. It is important to keep both muscles and ligaments strong if you want to keep your back in good condition. That is why exercise (which should include a varied number of movements) is so important. Bad habits at rest must also be avoided.

## That sudden pain

Almost everyone has experienced lower back pain at least once in their lives. The pain is usually severe, and in some cases so bad that it prevents you from moving. It can happen when you make a sudden movement, try to lift something heavy, or have been stuck in the same position for a long time. The muscles, tendons and ligaments in the back get overstretched, which leads to inflammation and swelling. You can also damage the discs so that they tear or stretch. If a disc breaks or is damaged (slipped disc), it will press on some of the nerves and cause pain. For example, if a disc is pressing on the sciatic nerve, which runs from the lower spine to the legs, it will cause pain that runs from your lower back all the way down your leg (this is called 'sciatica').

## First aid

When you get that sudden attack of back pain, lie down at once on the floor. Get on your back and hug your knees to your chest. Stay in this position until the worst pain eases. When you can move a little, still lying on your back, put your legs carefully on the seat of a chair with your knees bent. This way, your legs are at a 45° angle, and all the pressure is off your back. Try to rest like this for at least twenty minutes; then you should be able to get up and move about gently. Apply an ice pack (or bag of frozen peas) to the painful area and keep it there for twenty minutes.

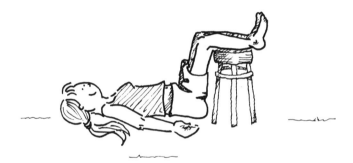

During the first few days, try to lie down on the floor in the position I just described (your legs at a 45° angle, your calves and feet on the seat of a chair) at regular intervals during the day. You should also take anti-inflammatory painkillers such as aspirin or ibobrufen to lessen the pain and thus make the muscles relax. Apply ice for twenty minutes several times a day.

## A pain in the neck

Many people also have recurring neck pain or stiffness in their upper back and shoulders. This is usually caused by strain or spasm of the neck muscles or inflammation of the neck joints. You could also have damaged the discs between the neck (cervical) vertebrae. Neck problems often cause headaches or pain in the shoulder, in the upper back or down the arm. This pain is sometimes related to tension in the trapezius muscles, which run from the back of the head across the back of the shoulder. It gives you a very tight and painful feeling.

If this happens to you, there are a few things you can do to relieve the pain. Back specialists often tell you to use ice for neck pain, but it could make you feel even stiffer. I find that heat is more soothing in this area. Soak a face-cloth in hot water and apply this to the back of the neck. A hot shower is also a good treatment, giving you a moist, hot massage. Try both ice and heat to find out which works best for you. Rolling your shoulders gently and turning the head slowly from side to side can help loosen the stiff muscles as well.

These self-help methods usually work well with mild pain and discomfort. If the pain is more severe, you must seek professional help, as neck stiffness is sometimes the first symptom of a serious illness.

*Call a doctor if:*
- ~ You have a stiff neck with a headache and fever
- ~ The pain extends down one arm or there is numbness or tingling in the arm
- ~ Lower back pain is accompanied by pain that radiates down one leg
- ~ You develop weakness in the arms or legs
- ~ A blow or injury to the neck (whiplash) has caused new pain
- ~ You are unable to manage the pain with home treatment

### People who can help you

It is important to see a back specialist if you have recurrent back pain. Your family doctor will refer you to either a physiotherapist, osteopath or chiropractor. They will assess your particular problem and teach you exercises that you can do at home. They will also look at the way you stand and sit, and show you how you can change bad habits. Exercise, massage or spinal manipulation is usually prescribed.

The *exercises* should be done daily because they will make your back strong and supple, reducing the risk of further injury. In addition to specific exercises for your back, you should also exercise in other ways, as a varied programme is the best way to ensure total fitness for your back. All-over strength means strong muscles in your abdomen, thighs and buttocks, which will greatly support the spine.

*Massage* of the muscles and tendons in the back is often very helpful. It can even be done by untrained persons, such as your partner, a member of the family or a friend. Some people have a special talent for this, and can give you a wonderful massage that will really improve the stiff and painful area. Good massage gives great relief and makes you feel supple. It makes it easier to exercise as well. The effect can last for days. If your partner, family and friends do not cooperate, you should seek professional help. A physiotherapist or licensed professional massage therapist will give you an excellent treatment. Regular massage (once or twice a week) may speed up your recovery considerably.

*Manipulation* of the spine has been used to treat back pain for more than a thousand years. (We did not start walking upright yesterday!) In this century, better techniques have led to the development of chiropractic and osteopathy. Spinal manipulation relieves pain by increasing the mobility between the vertebrae that are locked together or displaced. This way, trapped nerves are freed and the pain is reduced. The manipulations can range from gentle stretching or pressing to quite dramatic pulling and twisting; you sometimes even hear a loud cracking sound. You usually need a number of treatments to eliminate pain.

##  How to prevent back pain

Many back problems are a result of what you do while you are inactive rather than when you exercise. Standing, sitting and lying in bad positions are what cause most problems, which, more often than not, develop into chronic conditions. If you take little or no exercise, you are likely to have poor muscle-tone, with no strength to support your back. Adopting the wrong position is bad enough, but the fact that you often stay like this for prolonged periods makes it even worse.

## ❭ Good posture

Few people pay enough attention to their posture. It is something that should be taught to children at an early age, in order to make them have a correctly aligned back for life.

It is important to keep your back straight when sitting or standing. It not only benefits your back, but also ensures that your internal organs function properly. Bad posture can cause pinched nerves and other aches and pains. It can even interfere with proper breathing. Many women slouch in order to hide physical aspects they think are unattractive, such as a big bust, a spare tyre or (in their own eyes) excessive height. *Nothing looks worse than bad posture!* It gives the impression of poor self-confidence and lack of energy, and it can also make you look fatter than you really are.

Once you learn how to stand and walk correctly and make it into a habit, it will be completely natural. As I explained in Chapter 3, adopting the right posture is not difficult if you know how. Many people think that you should pull your shoulders back sharply, arch your back and lock your knees straight. This is incorrect. Starting from your knees and following through all the way to your head, correct alignment of the back means: your knees relaxed, your bottom pulled in, your waist pulled up, your shoulders relaxed (pull them up, then let them fall down to feel what I mean) and your head upright. Look at yourself sideways in a mirror to practise. Try to stand like this at all times. It will soon become a habit, and you will never again get tired from standing. You should always relax your shoulders. Aches and pains in the upper back and neck area are often the result of stiff shoulders.

If you are in the habit of carrying a heavy shoulder bag, you may have stiffness on only one side. Many women keep all they need for the day in such a bag. Keys, change, make-up, address books, diaries and mobile phones can weigh a ton when put all together in a bag. You probably lift your shoulder from time to time to keep your bag from slipping down, or keep it lifted for long periods. You must organise your load to make it lighter and carry your bag with the strap across your chest.

## Sitting properly

Many of you probably spend most of your day sitting down — at the office, in the car and on your living-room sofa. Sitting still for hours without paying much attention to how or what you sit on can give you back pain. It is all very well doing exercises for your back, but if you sit hunched over the computer at work and slouch on the sofa in the evenings, exercise will not make much difference: exercising for half an hour a day will not make up for slouching the rest of the time. Your furniture may look nice and suit your house. It reflects your taste and social status. You are probably very proud of your cosy sofa, attractive easy-chairs and big bed. But do they suit your back? Probably not. Most sofas invite you to slouch, many chairs force you to hold your spine in the wrong position and many beds are too soft.

Slumping when you are sitting can pinch the nerves in your back by pressing the muscles together. You should always sit upright with your buttocks all the way to the back of the chair. Place a cushion at the small of your back and relax your shoulders. Do not cross your legs. If you have a constant ache in your lower back, try putting a footstool under your feet. You can use a couple of phone books if you do not have a stool. This raises your knees slightly higher than your hips, relaxing the muscles in the lower back. Do not put your feet up on a chair or stool (or the coffee table) with straight legs, locking your knees. Many people like to sit like this without moving while watching television. This results in not only a stiff back, but stiff knees as well. Get up and walk around at regular intervals to loosen the back muscles, both at work and at home. You should never stay locked in the same position for longer than an hour or two. If you have to travel long distances in a car, remember to stop and walk around from time to time.

## Sleeping comfortably

Many people believe that beds should be as hard as possible to benefit your back. Although it is true that a soft mattress is bad because it gives little support and this puts extra stress on your back, a mattress that is too hard may prevent your muscles from relaxing. Your mattress should be firm and support your back comfortably. Placing a board under a too-soft mattress is a good short-term solution. Your mattress should be replaced every ten years or so, or earlier if it feels too soft.

If you have recurring pain in your neck and shoulders, it may be the pillows that are to blame, rather than the bed. Try a pillow made to fit the contours of the neck. These are now widely available in bedding shops and department stores. Too many pillows piled up under your head can put strain on your neck and shoulders.

The position you lie in also needs to be looked at. If you lie on your back, you may put strain on the small of your back. Many people have a hollow back, and lying in this way could then be the cause of the problem. If you must lie on your back, place a pillow under your knees. This will support your lower back and ease the pain. If you lie on your side, place the upper knee in the space behind the lower knee. If you are in pain, place a pillow between your thighs. This puts the upper leg level with your spine, taking the pressure off the nerves that are strained and irritated.

## Relieving stress

Stress can cause back pain, and back pain can, in turn, cause more stress. It may turn into a vicious circle that is hard to break. When you are stressed, you often tense your muscles, either in your shoulders or in your back. It may cause you to adopt the wrong posture or to walk stiffly. You may be completely unaware of this tension in your body, until you feel the pain. It is very important to break the circle of stress-pain-stress. Find out why you are so stressed, and try to think of a solution. Seek medical help if you have serious psychological problems in your life. It may be very helpful just to talk to someone about what is worrying you.

Having a massage or taking a sauna regularly may help to loosen stiff and tense muscles. Learning to relax by going to yoga or stretch classes is very beneficial. Once you learn how to relax your body, you will be able to release the tension. This may take a long time, but it will pay off in the end.

##  Your daily chores

It is important to pay attention to how you hold your back when you lift, carry and do other tasks which may damage your back. Housework, shopping and gardening can put a lot of strain on your back, shoulders and knees. *Lifting* is particularly risky, because most people do not realise that you also lift half your bodyweight when you bend over. When you lift something, be it heavy or light, you must bend your knees, keep your back straight and your feet apart. You should also remember to hold the object as close to your body as possible. Bending and twisting makes matters worse. Put the object straight in front of you, pick it up and move your feet instead of twisting before putting it down.

If you have to *carry* something really heavy, get somebody to help you. Sharing a heavy load between two people makes it easier. Never carry heavy shopping in just one bag. Share the load between two bags and carry one in each hand. This way you hold your back straight, the load is even and there is less strain.

If you have to lean forward while doing *housework*, always bend your knees. In the kitchen, open a cupboard and place one foot on the lowest shelf while preparing meals or washing up. Put one knee on the bed while you make it, instead of leaning forward with your knees locked. When you use the vacuum cleaner, keep your feet apart, knees bent and back straight.

Many women get back pain after *having a baby*. Your back is especially weak just after giving birth. When you are pregnant, your lower back and pelvic joints become looser in order to make the passage of the baby easier. In addition, looking after a new baby puts a lot of strain on your lower back. Perhaps you change the baby on a table, leaning over with your knees locked straight. Instead, change the baby on your bed, kneeling on the floor. When you bath the baby, put the baby-bath in the bathtub and kneel on the floor. Pay attention to how you lift and carry the baby, using the techniques I described above. Do not carry the baby around on your hip as many women do when the baby gets a little older. This twists the spine and puts a lot of strain on your lower back. When dressing small children, sit with the child on your lap, or put the child on a chair and kneel on the floor.

In the *garden*, be very careful of your back. Many people hurt their backs while gardening. Knees bent and back straight are two things you must keep in mind when you lift, dig, carry or push. Never twist your back while digging or raking. Move your feet instead of your back. In addition, alternate your grip when raking, digging or hoeing. Switch from the right hand to the left at regular intervals. Break gardening sessions into three-hour periods, rather than ten-hour marathons. Combine stretching with light gardening chores, such as 'lunge and weed': lunge forward with one leg, weed for about fifteen seconds, then change legs.

 ## Exercise

Years ago, doctors recommended several weeks of complete bed rest for acute back pain. In the last ten years, however, the approach has changed dramatically, and patients are told to return to their regular activities as quickly as possible. Research shows that most people with acute back pain do better when they rest briefly, return to their activities after a few days and start an exercise programme within two to four weeks. Inactivity is more harmful than rest when your back is hurting. If you do not move, your muscles become stiff and weak. Exercise makes your muscles strong, reduces swelling and improves the condition of your spinal discs. Patients are often told to exercise even if it hurts or feels uncomfortable. However, you should never do anything that causes *severe* pain.

When you are recovering from acute back pain, rest for a day or two and then go back to *gentle* exercise even if there is still some pain. Back specialists recommend working *through* the pain (unless you have pain all the way down the leg, which could mean a pinched nerve) because inactivity may lead to stiffness and more pain. Return to more vigorous exercise after two to three weeks.

Keeping physically active is the best way to ensure that your back stays in good condition. Taking part in sports or fitness classes regularly will keep your muscles strong and your ligaments and joints supple. Aerobic exercise (swimming, walking, jogging or cycling) is particularly good because it also helps overweight people lose excess weight. (If you weigh more than you should, you put extra strain on your back by forcing the spine into an exaggerated curve.) Avoid exercises that involve major bending or twisting (such as rowing and certain types of dance classes). Exercises such as yoga and stretching make you supple and improve the circulation in the muscles. A keep-fit class which includes movements where you arch the back as well as those that bend the body forward (without twisting and with your knees relaxed) and abdominal exercises, increases the strength in both muscles and ligaments. It is important, however, to tell the teacher if you have problems with your back.

Many back specialists prescribe a daily walking programme, especially for patients with chronic back pain. Walking improves the circulation and makes your thighs and hip joints more supple. It also increases the mobility in your back and makes your discs more elastic. Relaxing your shoulders and swinging your arms while you walk relaxes your neck and shoulder muscles and may help relieve pain in this area.

##  Back to normal

It is certainly possible to cure back pain for good. You have to examine everything you do in a normal day. Learn how to stand and sit. Be generally aware of your back at all times. Check your position regularly during the day, trying to remember the basic rules. It does not take long for good habits to become completely natural. You will soon align your back correctly without even thinking about it, mainly because it is more comfortable.

Taking care of your back can make the difference between an active and enjoyable life, and pain and misery that affects everything you do. If you have problems with your back, you are doing something wrong. Back pain never occurs without a reason. That is why learning how to align your body and taking regular exercise are the real key to solving the problems. If you do, you can finally say goodbye to back pain for good.

*Ten rules for a problem-free back*

~ Stand and sit correctly.

~ Get up and move around every hour, instead of staying stuck in the same position.

~ Bend your knees when you lift, and do not try to manage heavy loads on your own.

~ Never bend forward and twist at the same time.

~ Do not slouch in a chair or sofa while watching television.

~ Make sure your mattress is neither too soft nor too hard.

~ Relax your shoulders, and remind yourself to do this regularly.

~ Lose the extra pounds if you are overweight.

~ Be physically active by walking and taking other exercise regularly.

~ Learn to relax.

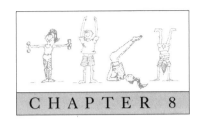

## CHAPTER 8

# CELLULITE IS ANOTHER NAME FOR FAT

The word cellulite was first mentioned in French medical literature in the early nineteenth century to describe female fat. It is not a disease, 'trapped toxins', an 'inflammation' or a 'condition'. It is simply fat, concentrated in areas where it is stored.

Fat is found throughout the body. It surrounds (as adipose tissue) all the internal organs and acts as a shock absorber. There is also a certain amount of fat under the skin. It protects us from pressure, shock and cold. Fat is important to the body in small amounts.

When the body has taken enough fat from the diet for its various needs, it stores the excess in one area, like a larder. Where your 'larder' is depends on your body type. Females are very good at storing fat. This is a talent they have kept since the beginning of the human race. Modern woman does not need this talent (nor does she wish to have it). Men store fat too, but they are not as good at it as women. Nor does their fat have the same composition. Most women store fat on the lower stomachs, hips, buttocks and thighs. Men usually have fat concentrated around the middle (the famous 'beer belly').

Female fat is different in its composition from the male variety. It tends to be lumpy and laid in perpendicular columns. Men have fat that is stored in a criss-cross pattern and this makes it appear smooth. Women also have thinner skin than men, which makes fat more visible. The type of fat found on the female body is harder to get rid of than that found on men. The reason for this difference is that in primeval times it was far more important for the females to keep their stored fat in order to sustain life for their young and to protect the reproductive organs. The human race survived because of cellulite! These days, we do not need to store much energy, as food is constantly available to most of us in the Western world.

Young girls do not, as a rule, have cellulite. It usually starts to appear around your mid-twenties, sometimes in connection with pregnancy. Most women have some cellulite. The fat on your thighs, bottom and stomach is usually dimpled and rough. Unevenness in your skin, which increases with age, adds to the lumpy look. It is increasingly harder to get rid of as you age. After forty, the body burns energy at a slower rate than before. The more overweight and inactive you are, the more cellulite you have. It cannot be completely removed, unless you were to lose all of your body fat, which would be life threatening.

##  A very female feature

Nothing is discussed more in the beauty sections of women's magazines than cellulite. It was a private problem before the early 1960s, when the fashion for the very slim, boyish figure started. Before then, women did have lumpy fat, but nobody got excited about it. A whole industry has grown up around it. It is astonishing that a bit of lumpy fat on women's thighs should cause so much anxiety and frustration. Women are made to feel that cellulite is a 'condition', nearly like an illness that must be treated and made to disappear. As with a number of beauty trends, businessmen in the cosmetics industry soon realised that they could cash in on women's need for the perfect figure.

Most women want to get rid of their cellulite, because they consider it unattractive. Many think that there is a miracle cure that will solve the problem. They are taken in by the pseudo-scientific mumbo-jumbo in advertisements designed to lure them into spending money on products that do not work. Fortunes have been made from this myth. Cellulite will not disappear simply by applying a cream. You can, however, greatly improve the appearance of cellulite with exercise.

##  What to do about it

I paid no attention to the whole issue until I was in my early thirties and living in France. Until then, I also thought cellulite was a disease. As I was in perfect health, I assumed it had nothing to do with me. I read about it in a French women's magazine at the hairdresser's. I learned how you get the 'orange peel effect' by taking a handful of flesh and squeezing. I could not wait to get home and squeeze, and yes, *I had it too*! Until then, I had been blissfully unaware of the problem. I decided to find the best method to get rid of it.

Fat can only be removed surgically or by burning it off while working your muscles. You can improve the appearance of areas with cellulite by exercising. Toned muscles squeeze the fat and make it look smoother. Aerobic exercise improves your circulation and makes you burn stored fat. Less stored fat means less cellulite.

Since the best way to improve cellulite is to remove the fat, aerobic exercise combined with a toning programme and a low-fat diet is the method to go for. The best aerobic exercise is walking, because it improves your circulation, increases your metabolism and tones the muscles in your thighs. Walking at a moderate pace is not too tiring, and this type of exercise forces the body to use stored fat without first using up the carbohydrate stores in your muscles (as explained in Chapter 2). If you have lumpy fat on your thighs and buttocks, walking regularly will gradually improve these areas. There is no exercise like it for firming your thighs (except maybe tap-dancing or step aerobics). Walking is available to everybody, without cost, equipment or a partner (even if it is more fun with a friend). You should walk for at least half an hour every day.

The areas affected by cellulite usually have bad circulation. Walking will also improve this. In addition, you can do leg exercises with or without weights. These improve muscle-tone and give you long, lean muscles very fast. When you work with weights, you can usually see an improvement even after three weeks. Most gyms have machines specifically for toning your legs. Some women have cellulite on their stomachs and even their arms. In that case, walking will still burn up the stored fat, and toning exercises will make the areas firmer.

As massage will improve the texture of your skin, you could try it as well. Use any cream that is quite oily. You have to massage vigorously for ten minutes every day. I find massage both pleasant and effective. It does not remove the fat but the skin looks smoother and more even. I have found that this, combined with walking and toning exercises, has made my cellulite virtually disappear.

## You are what you eat

Some magazine articles suggest that there are some foods that cause cellulite. It is said that certain foods contain 'toxins' (a fancy word for poison), which lodge in your fat stores and make it lumpy. Coffee, tea, sugar and chemicals in processed foods have often been blamed, as have even pesticides sprayed on fruit and vegetables. Although these things are not good for you, there is no medical evidence to support this theory.

You are often advised to drink a lot of water. It is good for your kidneys, your liver and, to a certain extent, your skin to drink lots of water, but there is no evidence that this will diminish cellulite. You should drink six glasses of water a day in addition to tea, coffee, fruit juice, milk and whatever else your daily liquid consumption contains. As water flushes out your kidneys more effectively than other liquids, it also helps prevent irritations in the urinary tract and bladder, which can lead to infections such as cystitis. It will not do anything to your fat stores, however.

It is also suggested that salt is responsible for water retention leading to cellulite. Retained water is not permanent and cannot cause fat to build up. Although too much salt is not good for you, it does little harm unless you suffer from a kidney complaint. Salt stimulates you to eat more, so it is wise to keep it to a minimum.

Sugar on its own is pure carbohydrate. Eating only sugar will, in principle, not cause you to put on weight. It is the combination of sugar and fat which is disastrous. The pancreas produces insulin to reduce blood sugar levels when you eat sugar. Insulin helps increase storage of fat. If there is no fat, there is no harm.

Unfortunately, most desserts, sweets and snacks combine fat with sugar. A sweet such as a meringue, which is made with sugar and egg white, is in itself not fattening. Put cream or chocolate sauce on top, and you have a dangerous combination! This combination is perceived by most people as irresistibly delicious. It is also highly addictive. Who hasn't opened a box of chocolates with the intention of having just one! It is far better to try to wean yourself off these treats. Learn to love fruit, which has lots of natural sugar. Fruit and vegetables contain vitamins and minerals that are essential for good health. They also have plenty of fibre which is important for keeping your digestive system healthy. Eating plenty of fruit and vegetables will improve your skin, making it smooth. If your cellulite is made worse by the fact that you are overweight, a diet low in fat will help.

##  Creams and lotions

'Smoother, slimmer thighs in a few weeks'! The advertisements in women's magazines sound so promising. The pictures of slim, young models with perfect, smooth thighs tempt you to try the products. These advertisements are particularly prominent during spring and early summer, when most women start thinking (and dreading the thought) of exposing their flesh in a swimsuit. What woman would not want thighs like that for the summer season? Especially if it can happen in a matter of weeks.

The advertisements are full of 'scientific' facts. It is said that the skin is 'drained', that the creams contain 'fat-reducing' agents, that they can 'reconstruct' the tissues and increase the metabolism of the skin. The marketing tries to make us believe in years of testing in laboratories and other 'medical tests'. It is maintained that women who have used these products have achieved wonderful results.

The French consumer magazine *Que Choisir* tested a number of creams and oils in 1997. Thirty women took part in this test. Half the group used one of the cellulite creams for a month, while the other half were given a normal cream without any 'reducing' ingredients. The result was the same for both groups. All women reported a reduction of 3 to 4 cm (about 1 inch). The skin was also smoother in all cases. This is quite a big reduction, when you consider that the average woman's thigh measures about 55 cm (22 inches).

The conclusion is that massaging *any* cream into your thighs will give a good result. Your blood circulation is improved by the massage and the skin is hydrated by the cream. It is as simple as that! These creams are pleasant to use and smell wonderful. They contain all sorts of weird and wonderful things. If you look at the lists of ingredients on the package, you discover a rich flora of mainly plant extracts: ivy, seaweed, algae, birch, cypress, horse chestnut and many others with Latin names. Some also list vitamins and caffeine among the ingredients. According to Swedish dermatologist Hans Rorsman at Lund Hospital (one of Sweden's biggest hospitals): 'cellulite and uneven skin is the result of a natural development. No cream or medication can change it.'

What is annoying about the advertisements is that they try to fool women into believing in an impossible dream. It is suggested that all the fat can be made to disappear. The creams are very expensive as well. The most expensive would come to nearly £200 for a litre. The average size of one tube is 150-200 ml, costing about £20. This amount lasts roughly two weeks, if you apply the product every day as you are instructed to. Most women would buy something like four tubes on average per season. The idea is that you must use them constantly to have a continued effect. This is true. But any cream works in this way (even olive oil). You have to keep massaging the areas for continued good results. As soon as you stop, your thighs will go back to the way they were before.

# Salon treatments

Beauty salons also advertise treatments for the removal of cellulite. They will submit you to all sorts of strange tortures in exchange for a substantial amount of your money. The treatments include the use of ultrasound, electric current and lymphatic drainage combined with pressure.

### Ultrasound

This treatment is said to make fat cells vibrate like an internal massage, causing fatty deposits to be 'naturally' removed through the body's lymphatic system. As if you could make fat disappear by 'vibrating' it!

### Electric current

It is claimed that fatty deposits are broken down by a four-stage twenty-minute treatment combining two types of current. A gel containing aminophylline (to stimulate 'cell metabolism') is used at home. You need ten to eighteen half-hour treatments.

### Lymphatic drainage with pressure

An even stranger treatment is one which claims to induce the removal of fatty deposits by lymphatic drainage. Aromatic oils are first applied to the legs, which are then encased in electronically operated, thigh-length boots that exert waves of pressure from foot to thigh (sounds like fun). It is recommended to have ten, and in some cases twenty, of these treatments, costing an average of £20 each. Many beauty salons use the term lymphatic drainage. They maintain that this type of massage, be it manual or with some sort of machine, will remove fat. This is false. As I said earlier, massage improves circulation which makes the skin smoother. It cannot reduce fat. (Try massaging a piece of bacon. Does the fat disappear?) It is recommended that you follow a diet while the treatment lasts. You will, of course, be slimmer at the end of the course, but probably as a result of the diet. Who is to know?

### ❱ Sticky bandages

Years ago, I tried something called 'Kwik Slim' (which was said to have a dramatic effect after only one treatment) to see if I could improve my thighs a little. It consisted of a sticky gel containing seaweed extract that was spread on the skin. My thighs were then wrapped in tight bandages which were left on for one hour. The result was sticky, but smooth skin. I was told by the person who measured me that I had 'lost' 1 cm (two-fifths of an inch) (probably from being squashed by the bandages for an hour). A few days later, my thighs were exactly as they had been before the treatment.

Assuming you have had a certain amount of success with one of these rather bizarre methods, it would be natural to think that you must go on using it to maintain the effect. Imagine the money you would have to part with!

##  Try electricity

There is a 'machine' powered by electricity that is supposed to help tone your thighs quickly. It has rubber pads that you stick on the offending areas. You then lie down on your bed or sofa, and the machine does all the work for you. The pads deliver mild electric impulses that contract your muscles. Each session takes twenty minutes.

These contraptions are often used by women who swear they have no time to exercise, yet spend hours on the sofa with electric pads stuck to various parts of their anatomy. It is hard to know if these things work. The models in the advertisements are always stick-thin both before and after. Muscles get strong when worked against resistance. In this case there is just an electric impulse: the muscle is made to twitch, not work. It will tone the muscles to a certain extent, but you do not get the beneficial effect that working the muscles yourself gives you, nor the feeling of well-being. As with the creams, it is not a magic cure for cellulite. If it really worked, it would be universally accepted, and no woman would have a speck of lumpy fat on her thighs.

##  How about a little surgery?

Fat removal by surgery was first performed in Argentina in 1958. The fat was removed from the patient's thighs and the long incision stitched up. It left ugly scars. Since then, techniques have improved, notably with the introduction of liposuction in the mid-1970s. This procedure involves vacuuming out the fat from the targeted area, through a short incision, leaving only a small scar. It can be used on either the stomach or the thighs. Some doctors even use this method to remove fat on the arms and under the chin. The patient is either put under general anaesthetic or heavily sedated. The incision is made at the natural crease of the skin on the area to be treated. A metal tube with several holes on one side is inserted and attached to a vacuum pump. The fat is then sucked out (ouch!). The area is tightly bandaged to prevent the accumulation of fluid, and the patient is sent home the same day. There is usually quite a lot of bruising and discomfort for about a week after the operation.

Liposuction can only be performed on slim people who are within 10 per cent of their target weight. Only the fatty deposits that are left after a weightloss programme can be removed (about 1 kg (2.2 pounds) maximum per thigh). Overweight women seeking this type of procedure are told to diet and exercise before they can be considered for the operation. The best results are achieved in women below the age of forty. After that age, the lack of elasticity in the skin makes the now empty area sag. A lifting and stitching of the skin is then necessary. This type of surgery is expensive. It costs about £3,000 for reducing the fat on the stomach, £2,000 for the thighs.

Liposuction does not remove the fat for good. If the patient gains weight again, new fat cells are created. The area becomes fat again, but this time with scars. (All that pain and expense for nothing!) It is especially important to watch what you eat and to take exercise afterwards to avoid this happening.

Liposuction has its advantages and disadvantages. On the plus side, it can dramatically change the shape of a woman who is carrying fat only on her thighs and lower stomach. It can also be used on the upper arms, but the result is generally not very good. On the minus side, there is a risk of unsightly and permanent darkening of the skin, unevenness and permanent scarring, and it is both expensive and painful.

##  Dos and don'ts

There are no quick-fix methods to get rid of cellulite. If you do not want to have surgery, a combination of diet, exercise and massage is the only solution. It may seem hard to stick to a routine at first, but perseverance really pays off. Here are a few dos and don'ts to help you:

**Do**
~ Walk for at least half an hour every day
~ Go for a longer walk (at least one hour) on Saturdays and Sundays
~ Follow the toning exercises shown at the end of this book at least three times a week
~ Massage the offending areas with a cream or oil after your shower. (Nivea makes a special lotion for massage which I find very pleasant to use.)
~ Eat less fat and more fruit and vegetables
~ Make this a permanent change

**Don't**

~ Sit around too much

~ Give up after a few weeks; patience and motivation are the two most important ingredients in a fitness programme

~ Worry if you slip up — you can start again; take it one day at a time

~ Make your weight fluctuate too much; constantly losing and gaining weight makes cellulite worse

#  Conclusion

As cellulite is (a) natural and (b) on most women, why worry? After all, it mostly affects parts of your body that are usually covered by clothes. You only expose your thighs to the public for a few weeks in the summer. Nowadays there are some nice, sheer wraps on sale to match most swimsuits. They look very pretty draped around your waist, and will hide most problems. In any case, other women on the beach or around the pool are probably too busy worrying about their own lumps and bumps to notice yours. Is there an Ideal Woman somewhere whose perfect body is the norm for how we should look? What a horrible thought!

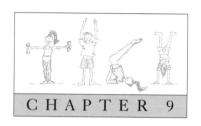

## CHAPTER 9

# MIDDLE-AGE DREAD

Menopause. This word has a ring of gloom around it. It is something women dread before it happens, avoid talking about while it does and will not admit to when it is over. The word itself conjures up images of an ageing body, a wrinkled face and horrible symptoms that you read about in the press. The menopause is not an illness. It simply means the ceasing of menstruation.

Perhaps women would fear it less if they were more informed. Most of them know that the menopause marks the end of their childbearing years. It is a bit like puberty, in that it is a landmark, but in reverse. When it starts and how long it will take varies from woman to woman. It can start as early as forty or as late as fifty-five. It is genetically linked. You will have a menopause very like that of your mother. There are certain symptoms associated with it that can be uncomfortable, embarrassing and sometimes hard to cope with. Many women see it as an end to youth and being attractive to the opposite sex.

Menopause was a taboo subject in our mothers' day. Occasionally, women would mention something called 'the change' to explain someone's odd behaviour or bad mood. Today, it is still not a favourite subject for discussion (you rarely hear it aired even at gatherings of the most broad-minded women). For many women, it is a sign of ageing, and very few want to admit that they have reached this stage in their lives.

Magazines aimed at the more mature woman are full of it though. Hot flushes, depression, fatigue, osteoporosis, dry skin. These are the negative aspects of the menopause that are constantly written about. You would be forgiven for believing that *all* women suffer from *all* these symptoms during their menopause. The truth is that it is a very individual experience and many women sail through it without much bother. Some do not have even the slightest hint of a hot flush or mood swing. Others suffer terribly. But if you look up the statistics, you will find that the figures are quite reassuring. While 75 to 80 per cent of women experience one or more symptoms, only about 30 per cent have severe symptoms.

## What happens during menopause?

During a woman's reproductive years, the pituitary gland, which is located at the base of the brain, produces the hormone FHS to stimulate the follicles in the ovaries to produce eggs, and also to produce oestrogen. Oestrogen builds up the membranes in the womb. Progesterone is then produced during ovulation. The womb is prepared for a possible pregnancy. If there is no pregnancy, levels of oestrogen and progesterone fall, and the lining of the womb, some blood and the unfertilised egg cell are shed. This is the bleeding that occurs each month. As you age, the number of eggs diminishes slowly. As a result, there is less and less oestrogen and progesterone. Your periods become more and more irregular, until they finally stop.

The menopausal process spans up to ten years, with most women having their last period around the age of forty-five to fifty-five. This hormonal imbalance can produce a range of symptoms such as hot flushes, night sweats, vaginal dryness, fatigue, migraines, urinary and bowel problems, anxiety attacks, depression and osteoporosis. This is a staggering list of ailments, but before you rush to the doctor for a dose of HRT (and to the pub for a large G & T), rest assured that many of these problems can be alleviated and in some cases prevented. Your lifestyle plays an important part in your health picture during this time. Research shows that you can help restore the balance of hormones through exercise and nutrition.

##  The hot flush

The hot flush is the best-known (and the most joked about) symptom of the menopause. Some 60 to 80 per cent of women suffer from it. It is the most common reason for seeking medical help. It feels like a sudden surge of heat that spreads through the body without previous warning. Your face becomes flushed and there is a sensation of heat mainly in your face and on your chest. This is often followed by profuse sweating. The thermostat of the body is disturbed by the body's hormone imbalance. It sets itself at a low temperature and the body reacts by overheating. If this happens at night, it can severely disturb your sleep. Sometimes you have to change both your nightwear and your sheets. If it happens during the day, you are worried that it will show. If you look at yourself in the mirror during a hot flush, you will see that it is not so dramatic. Your cheeks might get a little pink. The hot flushes continue for a few years.

### How to stay cool

A passive lifestyle makes the problem of hot flushes worse. Studies show that women who practise a lot of sports are relatively free from hot flushes. Activities that make you sweat (tennis, jogging or aerobics) improve the performance of your body's thermostat so that it is more evenly balanced. Vigorous exercise has also been proven to raise oestrogen levels in the body.

If you tend to get very uncomfortable, dress in layers, so you can remove clothes if you feel hot. Open the window, or keep a fan handy. At night, wear cotton nightclothes that are cooler on the skin.

Avoid too much alcohol, tea and coffee; these open the blood vessels and make you look flushed. Hot and spicy food should also be kept to a minimum. Try some of the soya products found in the shops. Soya has been proven to help, especially with the problem of hot flushes.

##  Depression, mood swings, anxiety attacks

The latest studies of the symptoms of the menopause indicate that the loss of oestrogen does not cause depression, as was previously believed. Women who suffer from depression or feel down during their menopause are usually reacting to real difficulties in their lives. This period in your life can be hard. Children leave home, you can have problems with elderly and ill parents, you may have to cope with the loss of loved ones. It is natural to feel sad and lost during such hardships. It is important to see these problems in their proper perspective and realise that it is normal to have low periods in your life, without blaming everything that is negative on the menopause. Many women who suffer from depression during the menopause have a previous history of this complaint.

### Exercise makes you happy

Nevertheless, some mood swings are associated with the menopause. It is similar to what happens during puberty. You feel emotional and tearful at times, but not to the extent of real depression. If you are mildly depressed, exercise should make you feel more positive and energetic. If your problems are more severe, you must seek help. See your doctor, who can advise you on therapy, counselling, medication and other ways to deal with it.

# Brittle bones

Your bones are constantly used up and rebuilt. It is a natural process. There is a gradual thinning of bone from the age of thirty onwards in normal people. With osteoporosis, more bone is broken down than rebuilt.

Osteoporosis in women has many different causes. The main factors are heredity and diminishing hormones. The time before and during the menopause is especially critical when it comes to osteoporosis. During this time bones can thin dramatically because of the decrease of oestrogen (which prevents bone-building calcium and protein from being lost from the bones and excreted in the urine). The first symptom is usually a loss of height. In later life there is a tendency for fractures, usually in the wrists, legs or spine. These fractures take a long time to heal.

It is a good idea to have a bone scan around the age of forty to forty-five, to measure the thickness of your bones in different parts of your body. This way you can find out if you are at risk, while there is still time to prevent it. Most hospitals have the equipment for bone-scanning these days. They measure your spine, hip joint and heel. You should ask your GP, who can give you the address of the nearest hospital with a bone-scanning service. Try in addition to find out if there is anybody in your family who has suffered from osteoporosis.

## Keeping your bones strong

It is encouraging to learn that there are plenty of things you can do to diminish and, in some cases, prevent the thinning of your bones. Weight-bearing activity is the type of exercise that is effective in the prevention of bone-loss. Anything that involves the body supporting its own weight on the ground is known as weight-bearing. Walking, jogging and aerobics (step aerobics, low-impact and high-impact aerobics) are the best examples. Cycling and swimming, although good for cardiovascular fitness, are not weight-bearing.

This type of exercise, combined with a diet rich in calcium, is the best recipe for strong bones. You need at least 800 mg of calcium a day before the menopause, and 1,500 mg after that. Three glasses of milk is about 800 mg. Eggs, cheese and yoghurt are also high in calcium. You do not have to worry about taking too much fat, because most dairy products are available in a low-fat variety. Low-fat milk products contain more calcium than the full-fat kinds.

There are many foods other than dairy products that have a high calcium content. Green vegetables such as spinach, cabbage, broccoli and many others are rich in both calcium and vitamins. You can also take calcium tablets. They can be bought over the counter at the chemist's.

The skin takes vitamin D from the sun, which helps the intestines absorb calcium. It is important to spend some time outdoors each day. You get plenty of vitamin D even on a cloudy day. Fifteen to twenty minutes a day is enough to benefit. Too much sun has an ageing effect on the skin, and also increases the risk of skin cancer; so be sensible.

Thinning of the bones is strongly associated with smoking, especially if you started smoking young and are a heavy smoker. If you stop smoking and in addition exercise and pay attention to your diet, this negative effect can be reversed. Brittle bones is only one of the dangers of cigarettes. The list of the risk factors of smoking is very long indeed. Make a serious effort to give it up: your health depends on it.

It is most beneficial if you start following these rules long before the menopause sets in, because you will then have the best chance of avoiding the thinning of your bones.

 ## Heart disease and women

Heart disease is the most common cause of death among menopausal and post-menopausal women. According to the British Medical Association, one in four women die of it in Britain and Ireland. It is far more common than breast cancer and other fatal illnesses. Nowadays, more women suffer from heart disease than ever before, due to a more stressful life, smoking and being overweight. A family history of high blood pressure and heart disease is an added risk.

Women of childbearing age rarely suffer from heart disease. Before the menopause, oestrogen has a protective effect. As levels of this hormone fall, there is a higher risk of heart disease due to a rise in blood pressure. Hormone replacement therapy protects you from rising blood pressure, as it replaces lost oestrogen. You should have your blood pressure checked regularly during the menopause. Exercise increases oestrogen levels in the body. A low-fat diet and regular exercise are the best ways to reduce blood pressure. A glass of wine a day is said to be beneficial to your heart and circulation as well.

##  Weight problems

The menopause is often blamed when a woman over forty puts on weight. The hormonal change during this time does not in itself cause you to get fatter. As you grow older, your metabolic rate slows down. That is why middle-aged people, both men and women, find it hard to stay slim. Middle-aged people tend to be less active than when they were younger. They also give in too readily to the pleasures of eating. Regular exercise speeds up the metabolism, which will make you burn fat faster. Toned muscles burn more fat than slack ones. That is an added reason to keep active.

Some women find that their body shape changes as they go through the menopause. Your body no longer needs to store fat around your reproductive organs because of diminishing female hormones. If you earlier had a pear-shaped figure, you may find that you start storing your surplus fat around the middle instead. Your previously slim waist may become thicker. It is up to you to make sure that fat has no chance to settle there, or anywhere else!

# HRT

The opinions of doctors vary when it comes to recommending hormone replacement therapy. Some doctors are very keen to prescribe it, while others are wary. The best thing is to read up on it in one of the many books on menopause found in bookshops today.

HRT is sometimes prescribed to women who complain of severe menopausal symptoms. It is a course of the female hormones, oestrogen and progesterone. It is given to replace a woman's own supply of these hormones when they are diminishing. The amount prescribed is based on a medical assessment. You take it either in pill form or with patches that are stuck on the skin. These patches are usually put on a small area of the skin, below the waist, where they deliver small doses of hormones; they are replaced every three or four days, using a different site each time. HRT gives you a level of hormones which is the same as before the menopause. This is said to keep you feeling well, but you no longer have a true menstrual cycle. There is a monthly bleed, but no ovulation and thus, no egg. Your womb simply behaves as if you are still producing eggs by building up and shedding the lining of the womb.

It is wrong to assume that you can continue an unhealthy lifestyle that includes smoking, high-fat foods and no exercise while on HRT. Hormones do not 'fix' your health. Whether you are on hormones or not, bad habits affect you in any case.

## HRT, for and against

**For**

*Generally*

HRT is beneficial to women who suffer from the many symptoms that come with the menopause; 90 per cent of women on HRT have reported an end to mood swings, hot flushes and sweating within three months. It also stops you putting on weight around the waist because you maintain the same level of hormones as before. HRT users also have thicker, more moist skin than non-users.

It makes your mucus membranes stronger and more elastic, increases muscle strength and makes you more energetic. It does not make you *look* younger or slimmer, nor does it mean that you do not have to make an effort to lead a healthy life, but it does make you feel better.

## Specific diseases

*Alzheimer's disease.* New studies have shown that HRT can protect against, or delay, the onset of Alzheimer's disease.

*Osteoporosis.* HRT stops bone-loss for as long as you take the treatment. It halves the risk of fractures after five years.

*Heart disease.* The risk of heart disease drops by nearly 50 per cent for the duration of the treatment. This is important for women with a family history of heart disease.

*Colon or liver cancer.* Recent studies have shown that HRT may reduce the risk of colon and liver cancer by nearly 40 per cent after ten years.

*Cataracts.* It has recently been suggested that women taking hormone treatments are less likely to develop cataracts.

## Against

*Generally*

The negative side-effects are unpleasant enough to make some women come off the treatment within the first year. These may include headaches, nausea, mood swings, tender breasts, erratic bleeding, weight-gain and skin rash.

### Specific diseases

*Breast cancer.* A woman's medical and family history plays an important part in the decision to use hormone therapy. If members of your family have had breast cancer, you should think twice about using hormones. The connection between breast cancer and HRT has not been confirmed, but the suspicion is there. It might be best to try to manage without it. Discuss this with your doctor, who will have the latest indications.

*Endometrial cancer.* HRT can aggravate conditions such as fibroids and endometriosis (thickening of the lining of the womb). The risk of cancer of the lining of the womb increases if oestrogen is used without progesterone (the hormone responsible for building up and later shedding, the lining of the womb during a woman's period).

### Coming off HRT

If you have been receiving HRT and want to stop the treatment, because of side-effects or other reasons, make sure that you stop gradually. Once you come off the hormones, you may experience the very symptoms you were trying to avoid. When you come off HRT, you will be at the stage you would have been without it. HRT does not bridge the gap between the pre- and post-menopausal stages. You should ask your doctor to wind down the dose over a few months to give your body a chance to adjust.

#  Natural remedies

HRT should not be the first resort if you start having menopausal symptoms. There are many natural remedies that may help you. It is best to try these first. Many of these remedies have benefits, other than that of balancing hormones, which you would not get with HRT. These natural ways to relieve menopausal symptoms include certain foods, homeopathy treatments, herbs and even acupuncture.

## ❯ Soya products and other foods

Soya products are known to have an effect on some menopausal symptoms, for example hot flushes. Women in China and Japan have virtually no menopausal symptoms, largely because of their high consumption of soya. (The Chinese do not even have a word for 'hot flush'.) It is said to be beneficial to drink two glasses of soya milk a day, which will also give a good supply of calcium. Recent studies also show that soya can reduce the risk of breast cancer by as much as 50 per cent. (Women in the East rarely get breast cancer.)

The same type of natural hormones are found in other plant foods such as green and yellow vegetables, rhubarb, almonds and linseed. Medical research shows that eating soya and linseed can reduce hot flushes, help increase bone mass and bring about other beneficial effects similar to those of HRT. Many nutritionists are knowledgeable about what food you should eat to get the maximum benefit from natural hormones. It is a good idea to get advice from one of these experts. There is also a book on the subject by Marion Davies, *Beat the Menopause Without HRT* (published by Headline).

## ❯ Homeopathy

You can also try homeopathy, which many women have found helpful. Homeopathic doctors treat women with menopausal symptoms by giving them small doses of natural hormones. Homeopathy works like a trigger to make the body produce its own hormones. The treatments are taken in pill form during three-week periods with pauses in between, in the same way as you would take a contraceptive pill. The doctor also prescribes additional remedies for some symptoms. Sulphur or sepia is recommended for hot flushes, natrum mur or pulsatilla for depression. You need to find a medical doctor who also practises homeopathy. Dr Andrew Lockie and Dr Nicola Geddes have written *The Women's Guide to Homeopathy* (published by Hamish Hamilton), which contains useful information about homeopathic remedies during menopause.

## Herbs

Some herbs contain substances called steroidal saponins, which act like hormones on the human body, very much as with homeopathy. Herbalism is a more simple form of treatment than homeopathy, using exclusively herbs in its remedies. The idea is to put the body on the right track, ending the treatment once the body starts working normally. The herbs include vitex agnus castus, false unicorn root, blue and black cohosh, hops and wild yam. Herbs are widely available, both in pharmacies and in health-food shops. Many people use herbs for different kinds of ailments and usually choose their own treatments. When it comes to treating menopausal symptoms, however, you should consult a herbalist. Only a specialised herbalist knows which herbs to use in this case. The herbs are prescribed on an individual basis, adjusting the treatment to your own specific needs.

## Acupuncture

Acupuncture is sometimes used to treat menopausal women. The acupuncturist also gives you a Chinese herbal remedy to take in addition to the acupuncture. The herbs are given as a result of tests to find out your individual needs. Acupuncture can improve your circulation and digestion and relieve both physical and mental changes that are associated with the menopause.

#  Do not let it ruin your life

The menopause is not an illness, but it can be a difficult time. You must seek help if you are having problems. Many women feel intimidated by doctors, who are often a bit dismissive of menopausal women. It is a time to be assertive and demand the right information from your doctor about treatments. Many doctors have their own pet projects when it comes to methods to relieve menopausal symptoms. It is up to you to ask about *all* the alternatives and to get informed. If you are not happy with the way you are treated, change to another doctor, until you find one that you are happy with. It is such a personal thing to talk about these kind of problems. If you feel awkward, it may just be that the relationship with your doctor is not quite right.

Even if you do not want HRT or any other treatment, it is still important to have regular check-ups. Many health problems that occur at this time can be successfully treated if they are discovered early.

 ## Ten important points about the menopause

1.  The severity of the menopausal symptoms depends on the rate at which your level of hormones fall. This is partly hereditary. If the hormone levels fall abruptly, you will have a more difficult time than if the process is quite slow. The same applies if you are coming off HRT. You must wind down the dose slowly.

2.  You benefit most from HRT if you wait a year or two after the menopause. That way, you will have fewer and less severe side-effects. If you wait until you have been free of periods for a year, you can go straight on to the type of treatment that does not produce a monthly bleed.

3.  Do not stop paying attention to family planning until a year after your last period. Before that, you may still ovulate while your periods are irregular. Pregnancies at this time are rare, but still possible. Late pregnancies carry a high risk for both mother and baby.

4.  If you have previously suffered from pre-menstrual tension, you may have difficulties during your menopause and you may experience side-effects if you take HRT. Try lower doses of hormones or one of the natural treatments.

5.  Side-effects from HRT can sometimes wear off after a few months. You have to be patient and stick to the treatment for a while. If you feel no better after three

months, go back to your doctor, who may try to lower the dose or change to a different product. The new vaginal gels may suit you better. As it is applied locally and in smaller doses, it is said to produce fewer side-effects.

6. Less-known menopausal symptoms include fatigue, palpitations, irritable bowel syndrome, headaches, confusion and irritability. These are more difficult to treat and should be dealt with one by one, because they may be a sign of something other than the menopause.

7. Fat stores in the body manufacture oestrogen. That is why thin women often suffer more from menopausal problems than women who are slightly chubby. Although being overweight is bad for your health, being too skinny also has its disadvantages.

8. The menopause affects the skin. It is even more important to protect your skin from the sun at this age than when you were younger. Although 95 per cent of all skin ageing is caused by sunlight, the loss of oestrogen means that your skin is less elastic, dryer and more sensitive than before.

9. The importance of exercise cannot be stressed enough. An active woman *does* have fewer problems during the menopause than her inactive friends. You will be more relaxed and sleep better if you exercise regularly. Many menopausal problems are aggravated by stress. Do yourself a favour and *move*!

10. A healthy diet need not be boring. Now is the time to start paying attention to what you eat. A low-fat diet will reduce weight problems and the risk of heart disease. Sufficient calcium ensures strong bones. Plenty of fruit and vegetables gives you important vitamins, minerals and fibre.

A new beginning

You learn as a teenager to accept and cope with puberty and all the changes it brings in your body. It is simply part of life. The menopause is the same thing, but in reverse. Learn to accentuate the positive. The fact that you can no longer have children might make you sad, but most women do not feel that they want to get pregnant at fifty. The end of periods is also positive. It cannot possibly be something you miss!

It is often a woman's perception of her menopause that decides how she is going to cope, rather like a pain threshold. If you have had many health problems in your life which may have involved great physical pain, you will probably not find that the symptoms of the menopause are as hard to bear. If, on the other hand, you have been lucky enough never to have had anything seriously wrong with you, menopausal problems could seem enormous. It also depends on your own life and how happy you are with it. You may have many problems at this time, which will make menopausal symptoms very hard to put up with.

This should be a liberating time, when you can at last think about yourself and what you want to do. It is never too late to take up a sport or learn something new. I know women who have gone back to school and even completed university degrees after their children have left. You must also take a good look at your lifestyle. Now is the time to improve it if you have not already done so. Flaws in the way you live affect you most during this stage. If you do not look after your health it can have a very negative effect on how you feel. You are the person who has the greatest influence on your physical and mental health. If you are informed about the menopause and what you can do to relieve symptoms, you will be able to take charge of your own well-being. A change in lifestyle could make you blossom. It should help you feel good and as a result make you look to the future with optimism. It is not the end of your youth — it is the beginning of a new life!

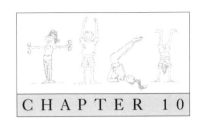

# SEXY AT SIXTY

Life does not start at forty. Nor does it end there. At forty, you should be in your prime. You often read in magazines that a woman is at her sexual peak around forty (just when your bottom starts to droop). The truth about that is hard to prove (though fun to try to find out!). The good news is that you can stay in your prime until well into your fifties and beyond — but it does take work.

The fact that you are getting older does not mean that you cannot have a good quality of life or that there is no pleasure left. Nor does it mean that you stop being attractive. It *is* possible to be fabulous at fifty, sexy at sixty, sensational at seventy, energetic at eighty, even naughty at ninety. It just takes some care and attention to health and more effort to keep up activities that you enjoy. In this chapter I explain what happens to your body as you age and how you can slow down the ageing process. I also show ways of staying youthful and attractive. Although you are no longer young, you can be stylish and elegant, with a great personality. The important quality in life is not to be young, but to be positive and fun to be with. You can be that at any age, provided you feel well and enjoy life.

# The ageing process

Theoretically, we start ageing from the moment of birth. But the first signs do not show until around the age of thirty-five. The way you age is partly genetic. It was thought until recently that 70 per cent of ageing was decided by genes. Recent studies show, however, that hereditary factors only account for 30 per cent of an older person's health picture. This proves that you are responsible for a large part of your health as you age. Let us look at what happens to the body at different ages.

## Twenty-five to forty

Between twenty-five and forty, your tendons and ligaments start losing their elasticity; at thirty-five your bones stop being built up and begin to thin. All your organs decline in quality. The impulses to your nerve cells slow down, and you no longer move as fast as when you were younger. Your breathing is not as effective as before, because your heart cannot pump at the same level of efficiency.

## Forty to fifty-five

Between forty and fifty-five, your brain begins to shrink and you start losing brain cells. Your metabolism slows down, so it is harder to stay slim. Your arteries and blood vessels start losing their elasticity, and the cells of your heart get weaker. Wrinkles get deeper and more noticeable because of a loss of elasticity in the skin, and the cells renew themselves more slowly. The force of gravity makes your breasts, stomach and bottom sag. The muscles of your eyes can no longer cope with seeing up close. You need glasses to read. The menopause starts at this age, with its annoying symptoms.

## Fifty-five to sixty-five

When you reach fifty-five, your skin gets even more wrinkled, your hair loses its pigment and goes grey, and age spots may appear. Your joints get stiffer and you no longer move with the same speed and suppleness as before.

### Seventy-five and beyond

After seventy-five, age-related illnesses and deterioration get more severe. Your muscle mass decreases by 30 to 50 per cent and your body is more bent and stiff. You find it harder to remember things. Your bones are thin, and injuries such as hip fractures are common among women. That is the bad news.

# The good news

Ageing is an inevitable part of life. You cannot stay young forever, but getting older does not have to be as bad as you may imagine. Both mind and body can be kept alert, fit and pain-free through a healthy lifestyle.

### Brain power

You can start losing brain cells as early as your thirties. That is why it is important to keep training your mind by doing things that make you use your brain. It is simply a matter of doing a little mental gymnastics such as reading, solving crossword puzzles or learning a language or a skill. Playing bridge and even bingo are excellent ways to keep the brain alert. Stimulating the brain does not only make it stay alert. It will continue to evolve. The more new experiences you have, the better it is for your brain. As long as your brain continues to be stimulated as much as possible, the connections (called neurons) between its different parts have a better chance of staying operational. If the brain cells are given a chance to stay active, the mature mind can appreciate the deep meaning to be found in life experiences. In this way, the mind enables you to see patterns and connections between different things. It is important to keep your curiosity and to continue to learn all through life.

### Heart, lungs and circulation

A healthy diet and plenty of exercise ensure that your heart is strong, that your arteries are elastic and free of cholesterol, and that your lungs work at their full capacity. Walking, swimming, cycling and other sports can be practised at any age. People who have kept active all their lives have a head start on their less active contemporaries. But it is never too late to start. You can take up moderate activities at any age, provided you are reasonably healthy. (If in doubt, consult your doctor before starting an activity you are not used to.)

## Staying strong and supple

The joints are designed to cope with the strain of weight-bearing and friction generated by the body's various movements through life. The bone surfaces in your joints are covered with a layer of cartilage, like a cushion. Synovial fluid provides lubrication. This fluid is produced by the inner lining of the capsule that surrounds and supports each individual joint. Years of use, misuse, disease, injury and infection can affect the joints.

Osteoarthritis is a part of growing old. Most people have some form of osteoarthritis as they age, though usually without ever showing any symptoms. The severity of its development depends on heredity and your lifestyle. It is mainly caused by excess strain (like any type of machine that is used too hard). Arthritis occurs mainly in joints that take the brunt of the body's weight-bearing and stress, such as the spine, hips and knees. In women, the thumbs, fingers and even toe joints are especially susceptible to arthritis, because women's joints in fingers and toes are finer than those of men. Because of the weaker female bone structure, an overweight woman is more likely to suffer from arthritis. The heavier you are, the greater the load your bones and joints have to carry.

If the joints are overworked in sports or through repetitive movements, they cannot cope and will deteriorate to some extent. Whereas exercising normally is good for you and even essential for good health, too much one-sided training will in the long run wear out your joints.

Swollen and painful joints should be rested. However, if there is only a little stiffness, gentle exercise will greatly improve the condition at an early stage, and even prevent it from getting worse. Stiff muscles and painful joints are not an inevitable part of getting older, as many people believe. Although women are more susceptible to arthritis than men, it is possible to stay supple and pain-free throughout your life. Having the right genes is important since the tendency to have joint problems is inherited, but a healthy diet and lifestyle can greatly reduce your chances of pain and stiffness.

Rheumatism is a condition that affects the tendons where they connect to the bone. (Tendons connect muscle to bone; ligaments connect bone to bone.) Inflammation at this location results in stiffness and pain, usually lasting for days and even weeks. If you have any type of severe pain, it is important to see a doctor. The doctor will diagnose the problem and refer you to a physiotherapist, who can then prescribe a programme of exercises to suit your particular needs.

Exercise induces stretching and strengthening of the muscles and joints. It also makes you more relaxed, which in turn reduces stress. Stress is often the cause of muscle tension and discomfort. If you are relaxed, it is easier to deal with chronic pain. If you keep active all your life, your muscles will be strong enough to support your joints, and your improved blood circulation will ensure elasticity and suppleness. It is up to each individual to keep the mechanics of their frame in good shape. (An aching and stiff body is definitely not sexy.) Your body is rather like a car; it has to be kept running smoothly and well oiled, without being driven into the ground.

## Muscle strength

The wonderful thing about muscles is that you can keep them strong as long as you live. You can also build up muscle strength whatever your age. Toned muscles are more efficient at burning fat, even at rest. Strength training, combined with weight-bearing exercise, helps to reduce osteoporosis. When the muscles are made to work, they tug on the bones and thus stimulate bone growth. Slack muscles are not attractive at any age. If you want to keep your looks, make sure that your muscles are well trained.

The type of training that you can do changes as you age. Even if you are no longer able to move with the same speed as when you were younger, it is still possible to maintain stamina. That is why older people can cope with long, slow activities, such as long-distance running. Cycling, walking, swimming and keep-fit classes are sports that older people can cope with and keep up indefinitely. Golf and tennis are other hobbies that many people continue to enjoy in later life. The most important thing to remember is that *you must not stop!*

##  Essential oils

The basic guidelines for a healthy diet are explained in Chapter 2, but there are some items that are especially important as you grow older. Many age-related discomforts can be relieved with the addition of certain minerals and vitamins. Omega-3 oils are one of the most important ingredients in an older person's diet. They can be used to treat, and even prevent, various diseases such as heart disease and rheumatoid arthritis. Omega-3 has also been proven to lower blood pressure, reduce arthritic joint pain and stiffness, and to relieve some skin diseases.

The oils are found in nuts, vegetables, linseed, walnuts, pulses, rape-seed, soya and oily fish. The type of omega-3 found in plant foods are not the type that the body can readily absorb. Oily fish, on the other hand, contain the type of oils that are quickly taken up in the body. Sardines, mackerel, herring, trout, tuna and salmon are all oily fish. Canned tuna does not contain much omega-3 oil, as it is cooked before it is canned. Pilchards and sardines are cooked in the can, so the oils are kept in. Two helpings of such fish a week should cover your needs.

Most people do not realise how important omega-3 oils are for good health, especially in later life. These oils would generally be described as fats. While too much fatty food can lead to health problems, some fats are vital for good health. These fats are called essential fatty acids and are included in the group of fats known as polyunsaturated fats (which are all good for you). Omega-3 oils were identified in 1929, when it was discovered that they are essential to the healthy development of the unborn baby, and to good health throughout life.

The Western diet of today is too low in omega-3 oils. (Except for Scandinavia, where there is a large consumption of herring in the form of 'Sill'.) If you do not like fish, you can take omega-3 in capsule form, which can be found at the chemist's. Cod liver oil is a good source of omega-3, but it also contains vitamins A and D, which are harmful if taken in too big a dose. It is best to take pure omega-3 in capsule form, or the new concentrated cod liver oils without vitamin A or D.

 ## Not just for babies

It is quite common for middle-aged and older people to think that they need no longer drink milk. On the contrary, dairy products are very important as you grow older. Since bones start to thin when you are in your thirties, your calcium intake has to increase from this age. Osteoporosis can be greatly relieved by a large amount of calcium, but it is important to take sufficient calcium even without the presence of this disease.

Many women give up drinking milk because they are afraid of putting on weight. But these days, nearly all dairy foods have a low-fat variety. If you have an allergy to dairy products, you can eat soya products, which are high in calcium (and also contain natural oestrogens which can relieve some menopausal symptoms). You should take 800-1,500 mg of calcium a day after the menopause. A glass of milk contains about 300 mg of calcium, one egg 52 mg, and one low-fat yoghurt 200 mg.

 ## Smoke signals

Despite the warnings from doctors and other health-care workers, smoking among women is on the increase. So is lung cancer, which was previously considered to be a man's disease. Women also smoke more heavily today than in the past. That means that they are coating their respiratory tracts from mouth to lungs with carcinogens (the substance that produces cancer) on average twenty times a day. Lung cancer is not the only disease you can get from smoking. There is also a risk of cancers of the cervix, larynx, oesophagus, bladder, pancreas, kidney and stomach. Smoking also causes strokes, emphysema, premature wrinkling, early menopause and a higher risk of ulcers and osteoporosis.

Women are genetically more vulnerable than men to the effects of tobacco. According to new research in America, women who smoke are three times more likely than their male counterparts to develop lung cancer. In addition, women who smoke and take HRT run an even greater risk of developing cancer.

Some women smoke to keep their weight down, and many are afraid that they will get fat if they stop. It is surprising that these women would prefer the risks of cancer and other fatal diseases to the relatively small health risk of a few extra pounds around their waist. Smoking speeds up your metabolism a little, and also curbs your appetite. The reason many people put on weight when they stop smoking is that they feel more hungry, and also that they have the habit of putting something in their mouths twenty times a day (the cigarette is usually replaced by sweets). This should not be a problem, if you pay attention to what you eat and take some exercise. Smoking is definitely not sexy. If you stop smoking, you will reduce the risk of contracting fatal illnesses, feel a lot better and improve the condition of your skin. Smoking is an addiction that is considered as strong as that of heroin. It is very difficult to give it up. If you are having problems, consult your doctor, who may prescribe nicotine chewing gum, or recommend hypnotic treatment or acupuncture. If you really want to give up smoking, you will succeed.

Do yourself a favour, stop smoking today!

#  A lovely complexion

The skin is the body's largest organ. In an adult, it measures about 2 square metres (7 square feet). The skin regulates the temperature of the body by sweating and by opening and closing the pores. It protects the body from harmful toxic substances and the rays of the sun. Bacteria and viruses are eliminated by glandular secretions. The skin also acts as an antenna. Stimulation from outside, such as cold, heat and pain, is felt by the nerve endings, and signals are then transmitted to the brain. The skin shows signs of ill-health and the symptoms of some illnesses by producing rashes and redness. A very pale skin is the sign of ill-health. Your skin is at its best when you look after your health.

You should take good care of your skin. It is said that when you are young, you have the skin you were born with, and as you age, the skin you deserve. There is a lot of truth in this, since you can damage your skin by the way you live. If you smoke and spend a lot of time sunbathing, your skin will age prematurely.

Some 95 per cent of skin ageing is due to sun damage. The only woman I ever met who had never overexposed her face to the sun was my grandmother. She had lovely, youthful skin even at eighty, so it must be true. (She was not what you would call thin, which also helped plump out her skin.) Unfortunately, by the time I paid any attention to what she said, I was already in my forties and had spent many wonderful holidays in the sun. My skin would probably be a lot better if I had followed her example.

These days, the bad effects of the sun are widely known, but most women still like to have a tan in the summer. The creams for suntanning are now highly protective and most people are aware of how to use the different protection factors. Even so, most dermatologists would prefer that you stay out of the sun altogether, as there is still a high risk of skin cancer even while using protective creams, due to the thinning of the ozone layer.

Doctors maintain that most people do not put on a sufficiently thick layer of cream, and that they do not renew applications often enough after swimming. There is also a tendency to stay out in the sun too long because of the false sense of security the creams bring. Older people benefit from small amounts of sunshine, which gives them the vitamin D they need for strong bones. Fifteen minutes a day is sufficient, however, and the time in the sun should be in the morning or evening, thus avoiding the strong midday sun.

Sunbeds, which were previously thought to be a healthier way to get a tan, are now considered to be as dangerous as the real thing. A recent report by the Health Education Authority in Britain says that people who use sunbeds regularly increase the risk of skin cancer. A tan from a sunbed gives no protection from getting sunburned.

Women's magazines are trying their best to promote a pale look, to prevent women from spending too many hours in the sun. They inform you of the damaging effects of sunlight and the increased risk of skin cancer. The fashion models of today look a lot whiter than they used to, even when showing summer clothes. Hopefully, women will start to realise that brown skin is not a sign of good health, but of damaged skin. Fit people look healthy even when they are not tanned, because of good blood circulation.

If you insist on being brown in the summer, you can either use a fake tanning cream or lotion (which will give you a 'tan' in a few hours), or apply a tinted cream. Imagine how much free time you will have if you decide to simply stay white!

##  Wonder creams

There are many creams, oils, lotions and potions on the market today that promise near miracles in the reduction of wrinkles. The more expensive they are, the more they promise. You would need a degree in chemistry to understand some of the advertisements. You could get totally confused reading about ceramides, liposomes, collagen and AHAs (alpha hydroxy acid), to name only a few of the magic ingredients. Your daily ablutions are becoming more and more complicated. You are supposed to cleanse, moisturise, tone and exfoliate, though not necessarily in that order. All this takes a lot of time, energy and hot water: the rest of the family may also want to use the bathroom occasionally!

It would be wonderful if you could turn the clock back and undo the damage of time simply by applying a cream. Unfortunately, that is not possible. According to dermatologists, no cream can make wrinkles disappear. You can prevent them by not sunbathing or smoking, but once the damage is done there is no going back.

##  The moisture trap

What makes skin soft and smooth is mainly water: therefore the more water you can keep in your skin, the better you look. If you use a good moisturiser daily, your skin will keep its softness. The cheaper creams sold at the supermarket are just as good as the expensive ones, and they contain sun-protection factors as well. (Ultraviolet rays can age your skin even during the winter months.) Doctors even say that Vaseline will do the job just as well as any of the more expensive creams.

Creams containing vitamin E are said to have a beneficial effect on ageing skin. The expensive creams are lovely to use, and usually smell wonderfully of various perfumes. There is nothing wrong with using them, if you can afford to. It gives you a wonderful feeling of luxury to smother an expensive product on your skin. Do not expect miracles, though!

##  Nip and tuck

Women approaching fifty often start thinking of cosmetic surgery. You probably know at least one woman who has had some kind of surgery. You may even have had something done yourself. Plastic surgery is becoming more advanced and more widely available. If the result is good, you will have smoother skin and a more youthful appearance. Some women are delighted with the result of their whole or partial face-lift, but others are very disappointed.

A face-lift does not stop the clock. Your face will continue to age with time. You may have to repeat the procedure five or ten years later. You certainly will have smoother skin after just one face-lift, but it seems a very traumatic experience to go through simply to have smooth skin.

 # Less aggressive methods

There are several alternatives to a full face-lift. These treatments are done either in the surgery of a skin specialist or at a beauty salon. The methods include chemical peeling, ultrasound and injections of collagen and other substances under the skin.

### Chemical peeling

Peeling was performed only by dermatologists until quite recently. Through peeling, skin that was coarse, wrinkled and sun damaged became smooth and young looking again. (But it did not make sagging skin tighter.) The healing period, however, was long and painful. There is now a more gentle variation of this, which is used by trained skin therapists. Called Doctor Dermatologic Peeling, it involves stripping the upper layers of the skin with acids. Just after the procedure the skin looks white and 'frosty'. Later it starts to feel hot, and to seep and redden. After a few days it starts to peel. Finally, the new skin appears, soft and smooth. The new skin is very sensitive to make-up, water and perfume. You must avoid sunlight afterwards. The treatment costs about £500.

### Ultrasound

This treatment involves the use of ultrasound (called Sonolift) to make a moisturising gel penetrate to the deeper layers of your skin. It is supposed to stimulate the production of collagen and elastine in the skin, which make it more supple and elastic. This treatment has had a lot of success in France, where women are very enthusiastic about the results.

## ) Injections

There are also several different types of injections for treating the skin. Some use collagen or a product called Artecoll, which is made up of microscopic glass-fibre balls. This substance is inactive and does not give allergic reactions. Artecoll also contains collagen, which is a natural substance. When the product is injected under the skin, the body's own tissues build a 'shell' around it. This fills out the wrinkles. The results are long lasting, and apart from small correction in some cases, stay in your skin for many years. This method works best on deep wrinkles, such as those that can occur between the eyes and below the nose. Many women say they look and feel ten years younger after the injections.

Dermatologists in Sweden use a method where the wrinkles are injected with Restylane, which is a chemically produced acid like that which is naturally present in the skin when you are young. You gradually lose this substance as you age and your skin gets less elastic. The results of this method are excellent, but the effects disappear after about six months. You have to renew the treatment at regular intervals. The same applies to injection with collagen.

Finally, there is lymphatic drainage of the face, which is a type of massage with suction cups, and Mini wrinkle tone, which is described as 'aerobics' for the face; it is said to stimulate the facial muscles.

There are many other methods. They are constantly advertised in the press, and the before-and-after treatments look very impressive. It is up to you to decide which, if any, you want to try.

Looking older is one of the facts of life that you have to accept. If you have the courage to face the world as an older woman, you will fare better than if you are constantly trying to pull your face about in the quest for a youthful appearance. If you look after your health, you will enjoy life to the full, even if your face is lined and your hair grey. It is the happy look in your eyes that makes you look attractive.

#  Looking good

It takes a lot more effort to look attractive when you are older. A young woman simply needs a little lipstick and blush to enhance her looks. The more mature woman has to spend a certain amount of time and money on her hair, skin and clothes in order to look well groomed and attractive.

## ❭ Your hair

No woman needs to have grey hair. You can dye your hair any colour you want. It can be done either at home or in a hairdresser's. You get the best result at the hairdresser's, where great care and attention are paid to getting the colour right without damaging your hair. A good hairdresser will also advise you on the best shade for you.

A good cut is important for the mature woman. Long hair is not attractive on the older woman, but well-cut hair can be most becoming. It is the one thing that can improve your looks the most. Even grey or white hair can look wonderful if you have a good cut. There is no need to dye your hair if you prefer keeping your natural colour.

## ❭ Make-up

The older woman needs to wear a little make-up to even out skin tone and to add colour. It is a good idea to go to a beauty salon for advice on the type of make-up that suits your individual needs. Many department stores also offer a free make-up session to try some of the different makes on the market. (They would like you to buy the products after the make-up session, but you are not obliged to do so if you are not happy.)

Remember, less is more when it comes to make-up for the mature woman. Too much make-up of the wrong kind can look ageing instead of giving the younger effect that you were trying to achieve.

## ❯ Dressing up

There is great equality across the ages these days. Older women now wear clothes that were previously thought to suit only younger women. Everybody wears jeans, T-shirts, short skirts and even Bermuda shorts. Women no longer have to give up the styles they prefer because they are a certain age. The way you dress reflects your personality. If yours is flamboyant and colourful, go for it!

The colours that suit you change as you get older. Your hair, skin and eyes usually turn a paler shade, so you may have to change the colours that you wear accordingly. Many older women look better in pastel shades, which they may not previously have considered.

*If you want to be sexy at sixty, you must:*

~ Take plenty of exercise

~ Have a healthy diet

~ Not smoke

~ Look after your hair, making sure it is always well cut and conditioned

~ Stay out of the sun. (Even if you have wrinkles, avoiding the sun from now on will ensure that they do not get worse.)

~ Use a good moisturiser

~ Find out which make-up suits you best and learn how to apply it

~ Wear good quality underwear

~ Choose clothes that flatter your figure and that you are happy to wear

~ Consider changing the colour scheme of your clothes

#  Do not act your age

All the negative effects of ageing may seem depressing. Your body and mind go downhill. The future seems very bleak indeed. It is reassuring to learn, however, that there is so much you can do yourself to make sure that you age well. You can even have better health than people who are much younger. A seventy-year-old person who has kept active all her life has better health than someone half her age who has not.

Your body was made for movement. Keeping physically active is the best way to ensure that the ageing process does not ruin your life. Old people who take part in fitness programmes and vigorous sports are not freaks of nature. An eighty-year-old who swims fifty laps a day or walks five miles to the post office is not unusually vigorous. It is quite normal to be able to do things like that even if you are old. Everybody can achieve a good level of fitness at an advanced age, provided they have good health. Older people can now not only live longer than ever before — they can also have fun and feel happy at any age. The party does not have to be over at forty!

People who achieve great things or look amazingly good at an older age are now admired and applauded. Looking good and being fit should be the rule rather than the exception. It *does* take a lot of self-discipline to keep yourself looking well and to stay fit when you are older. It is hard and sometimes even painful, but the rewards are well worth the effort. It is surprising how active you can be well into old age. It is often a person's own perception of what she can do that slows down her physical activity. That is why it is important to forget your age and concentrate on how you feel instead.

Nobody knows how long they are going to live, but it is possible to have a good quality of life as long as it lasts. It is more important to put life into your years, than years into your life.

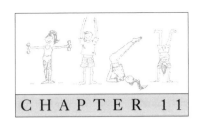

## CHAPTER 11

# LET YOURSELF GO

**M**odern life is becoming more and more stressful, especially for women. If you work full time, take care of children and do most of the housework, there will be a considerable amount of stress in your life. As you grow older, you find yourself with teenage children, who still need a lot of love and attention, and often, elderly parents. You may also have financial problems, with a mortgage, bank loan, school fees and so on. It is important to keep healthy, if you are to cope with such a lifestyle. A certain amount of stress is good for you. If there were no challenges in your life, you would soon get bored, and even depressed.

The amount of stress you can cope with depends on your personality. Indeed, some people even seek it in pursuits such as hang-gliding, parachuting, mountaineering and other dangerous sports. That sort of stress is very stimulating. Negative stress, however, can seriously affect your health. It can cause high blood pressure, cardiovascular disease and increased cholesterol. If you are very tense, you may develop back pain and other muscular problems. Long-term stress affects the immune system, making you more susceptible to colds, flu and other more serious diseases.

Coping with stress

### Exercise and stress

Aerobic exercise is one of the most effective ways of reducing stress. It lowers blood pressure, increases cardiovascular fitness, improves muscle-tone and triggers the release of endorphins (the hormones that give you a feeling of well-being). Regular exercise increases your energy, improves your memory and concentration, boosts your immune system and gives you better self-confidence. In short, exercise helps you cope with life.

### Taking time off for yourself

Learning to relax and take a break is an essential part of stress management. It is important to think of yourself from time to time. Women spend so much time looking after the needs of others and forget to make space for themselves. It is very good for your feeling of well-being to take time to look after yourself, preferably doing something that you enjoy. You must also try not to expect too much of yourself. Stop looking only at the negative aspects and discover the positive ones.

If you do something you enjoy at least once a day, it will lower stress and improve your immune system. If you feel positive and happy, you are more likely to be healthy and live longer. Several studies support the view that you probably held anyway: being negative is bad for you. The things that you enjoy could be anything at all: chatting to a friend, listening to music, being creative by making something, or cooking. It works as long as it brings you joy.

#  Being happy keeps you young

Bad mood sends negative signals to the part of the brain that controls important systems such as your immune and cardiovascular systems. In 1973, a German psychologist, Dr Ronald Grossart-Maticek, began a study involving some 3,000 residents of Heidelberg in their early sixties. He asked them what gave them pleasure and how often they did something they enjoyed. When he returned twenty years later, he found that the people who had been the most positive and happy were up to thirty times more likely to be alive.

The younger you are, the easier it is to get pleasure out of life and have a good attitude to it. You can, however, train yourself to think positively. You just have to get rid of the notion that enjoying yourself is somehow wrong or sinful. Women have a much greater tendency to think like this than men. You have to be more assertive when it comes to taking time off just for yourself. Get somebody else to mind the children, do the shopping, hoover the dog, or whatever it might be. Establish certain times of the week as time off for yourself, and treat these as being just as important as anybody else's time off.

You may enjoy learning something new, such as a foreign language or furniture restoration. Going to a class once a week is relaxing and enriching. You will make new friends who share your interests. It also gives you a special moment, in an otherwise busy life, to think only of yourself. You will, for that short time, not be somebody's mother or partner, but yourself. This 'breathing space' will help you cope with having to constantly think of your family's needs. It could get you out of bad habits like 'comfort eating' or sitting passively in front of the television watching rubbish.

If you can improve the quality of your life, it will be better for everyone around you. You will be happier, more positive and easier to live with. This might come as a great surprise to your loved ones, especially if you were previously a grouch. It might even make them feel slightly nervous. Just tell them that this is the new you, and that she is here to stay, as long as she gets what she deserves. A bit of blackmail can work wonders!

##  Lighten your load

Most women have a daily agenda that is packed with appointments. There is work, doctor's appointments, children's activities, and maybe community projects. Few women fit in something for themselves. Try to change this by taking an empty page in your diary a few weeks ahead and book time for you first. It may seem silly to write down things like 'take a walk' or 'read a book' at first, but it will soon seem normal. Just writing down words like 'fitness class' or 'yoga' will help you keep these dates and remind you of the importance of looking after your own well-being as well as that of others.

When you feel most stressed out, make a list of all the things you think you have to do. Then sort out what is most urgent, and what is not. This way you have a clear picture of what is most important. You may even find that you can remove some things off the list. It is guaranteed to save you having a panic attack. Reducing the list by even one item will make you feel instantly less pressured.

##  Split your day into sections

This works for me. When I have more things on my plate than time, I split the day into time zones. I say: in half an hour I will have done task x. I concentrate on that half-hour and nothing else. I do not worry about the rest of the day: the only thing that exists in my mind is my task and the thirty minutes ahead. When the half-hour is up, I take a short break and after that, another half-hour and the next task. I also make myself stop when the time I have allotted to my work is up, even if I have not managed to finish everything I set out to do. This method helps me organise my work more efficiently and I feel much more in control.

##  Simplify grooming

You can still look your best even if you take a few shortcuts in your daily beauty routine. Get your hair cut in a short, manageable style. Use shampoo and conditioner in one. A tinted moisturiser, blush and mascara should be enough for any woman on a normal working day. Pare down your working wardrobe to a few favourite outfits in matching colours. Take out the outfits you normally wear to work and sew on missing buttons, repair torn hems and other minor faults. Have anything slightly grubby dry-cleaned. This way you will have a working wardrobe and no last-minute panics that make you miss the bus.

##  Give a party

You may think this sounds crazy, but many women have little or no social life because of their heavy schedule. Seeing your friends and laughing with them gives you a break from your everyday routine. A party need not be hard work if you get some friends (those you still have left) together and make everybody bring some food. Start a new fashion: the pot-luck supper. Your friends will dare to give one themselves, and before you know it, you will have a social life again without much effort.

##  Bathroom bliss

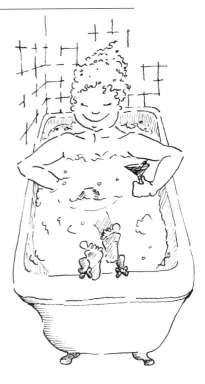

One evening a week, tell the world to go away, and turn your bathroom into a beauty salon. Wash your hair, apply a conditioning treatment, wrap your hair in a towel and take a long, relaxing bath with some nice-smelling bath oil. Listen to music while you relax. Apply a face mask that you leave on while in the bath.

Afterwards, dry yourself vigorously and apply body lotion all over. Remove the face mask and put on some moisturiser. Give yourself a manicure and a pedicure. Dry your hair and go to bed with a good book. You will not have too much trouble falling asleep.

If you work at home and your children go to school, this moment could take place in the morning, when everybody has left, after your walk or exercise session. It is *not* wrong, frivolous or selfish to spend a little time looking after your body. You will look and feel *wonderful* if you do.

#  The rest of your life

A good night's sleep is essential. It makes you feel rested and ready to face the day. Getting your 'beauty sleep' is increasingly important as you grow older. No amount of make-up can hide the effects of a bad night's sleep on your face. Fatigue will also affect your performance at work and make you irritable at home. Sleep is important for both the brain and the body. It gives the body a chance to rest and recover from daily activities and, more importantly, your brain re-sorts and stores information and 'recharges its batteries' while you sleep.

There are five stages of sleep: drowsiness, light sleep, deep sleep, deep/slow wave sleep, and REM (dream) sleep. Each one is important for the body for various reasons. That is why you need up to eight hours' sleep. Any less than that, and you will feel tired the next day. Alcohol and sleeping tablets may make you sleep for the required number of hours, but they affect the quality of your sleep, because they stop you from going through the important stage of dreaming. That is why you never feel as rested after taking sleeping pills. Alcohol may make you go to sleep, but you wake up a few hours later, and are then unable to go back to sleep.

Unfortunately, problems with falling asleep or staying awake for hours during the night are all too common. Stress, worry, pain and discomfort can disturb your sleep. As you get older, you are more easily awoken by noise.

### Sleeping repairs the skin

New research shows that the body repairs itself during the night. This is most noticeable on the skin. That is why you may go to bed with a spot on your face, and find it gone in the morning. The skin also absorbs helpful ingredients in creams most efficiently while you sleep. You should apply a richer cream in the evening than during the day. The latest night creams contain sleep-inducing essential oils, such as valerian and lavender, to help you achieve a good night's sleep.

## Insomnia and its causes

The main causes of insomnia are anxiety, stress, tension, depression, indigestion and pain. You can upset your body clock by, for example, staying up too late or going on a long-distance flight (jet lag). You can also get into a vicious circle, where the fear of not being able to sleep keeps you awake. Middle-aged women often have sleep problems because they are still 'programmed' to listen to small children waking up, rather like shift workers who suffer from insomnia up to ten years after ending their shift work. A healthy sleep pattern is easily upset, and difficult to get back to if something disturbs it.

## A snooze by any other name

A nap, snooze or siesta in the middle of the day used to be something many people enjoyed but were embarrassed to admit to. This is now called a 'power nap' and is recommended to busy executives to cope better with the demands of a stressful day (and to make up for lost sleep). Even if you are not an executive, you can still benefit from a short rest in the middle of the day. Many people feel sleepy around 2 p.m. There is a natural reduction in most people's body temperature around this time, which accounts for the drowsiness. A short nap of fifteen to thirty minutes is very refreshing, but if you sleep longer, your sleep will be too deep, and this will make you more tired when you wake up.

## Make your bedroom an oasis of peace and tranquillity

The room you sleep in should be a no-stress zone. Ban televisions, radios, computers and even the telephone from your bedroom. With the exception of something to play soft music on, your bedroom should be 'gadget-free' and should be the place you unwind and relax. Scatter pillows on the bed and strew around scented candles, pot-pourri, plants, favourite photos and books. Make sure the lighting is soft and free of glare. This way you will feel instant peace and calm when you rest.

*Helpful hints for a good night*

~ Go for a short walk before going to bed.

~ Go to bed at the same time every night.

~ Avoid coffee, tea and alcohol just before sleeping: have a cup of herbal tea or a glass of milk.

~ Have a bed-time routine, which may include having a warm bath, reading a book or listening to soothing music.

~ Use relaxing essential oils, such as lavender, either in your bath, or on your pillow (a few drops is enough).

~ Take some kind of vigorous exercise during the day, but not too close to bed-time. People who exercise regularly have normally few problems sleeping. Exercise within two hours of going to bed may make you too alert to sleep.

~ Do not watch television in bed. It can make you too wide-awake at a time when you should relax.

~ Make sure your bedroom is neither too hot nor too cold. It is easier to sleep in a cool bedroom. It should also be dark, as light stimulates the brain and keeps you awake.

~ If you are still awake after an hour, or you wake up and stay awake after a few hours, put on the light and read for a while, or get up and do something else. (How about some ironing — that should put you to sleep in no time!)

~ If you suffer from serious, chronic insomnia, consult your doctor.

# Conclusion

'Letting yourself go' a little from time to time is good for you. It makes life easier to cope with and gives you enough energy and enthusiasm for your daily life. If you constantly have to think of others, being a little selfish at certain times will make you a better mother, partner, companion, friend and co-worker. You will feel happier and more positive, which can only be of benefit to the people around you. You have the right to some time off, make sure you get it!

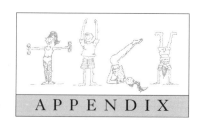

# THE BUSY WOMAN'S TONING PROGRAMME

This programme takes fifteen minutes to do. Start with just a few repetitions in the beginning and work up to the full amount. Put on some music with a good, lively rhythm to make it more fun. Try doing it in the morning, especially if you have problems with your back. It is a great way to start the day!

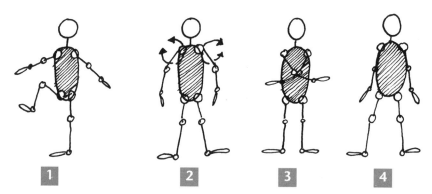

1. **Warm-up**: Walk on the spot for two minutes, swinging your arms.
2. **Shoulder roll**: Standing with legs apart, roll your shoulders to the back ten times and to the front ten times.
3. **Bust toner**: Arms straight in front shoulder level, twenty scissors.
4. **Waist toner**: (Pay extra attention to correct posture here!) Stand with feet apart, *knees relaxed, bottom in*. Pull up from the waist and relax your shoulders.

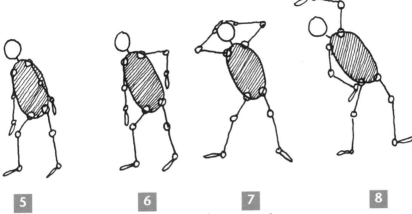

**5**  **6**  **7**  **8**

5. Bend down right side to touch your knee, ten times.

6. Repeat, but this time bend your elbow on opposite side. Ten times.

7. Put your hands behind your head and bend to right side, ten times.

8. One hand just below your hip, the other arm over your head, ten waist bends.

**Repeat exercises 5-8 on the left side.**

9. Bend your knees and keep your bottom tucked under. Pull up at the waist, relax your shoulders. In that position (with the knees bent), hold your hands together in front of you, and turn to the right ten times, then the left ten times. Repeat. *Do not move your hips!*

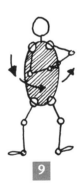

**9**

 ## Abdominals

10. Lie on the floor with your knees bent and your feet flat on the floor hip-distance apart, arms down by your sides.

11. Roll your head and shoulders up and try to touch your heels. Do four sets of ten.

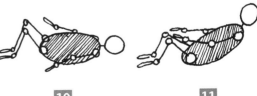

**10**  **11**

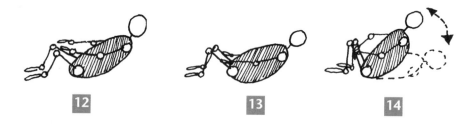

12. In the same position, touch the outside of one knee with both hands twenty times, then the other knee twenty times.

13. Still in the same position, roll up, grab your thighs and then **14.** pull up and down ten times, bending and straightening your elbows. Release and repeat. Do four sets of ten.

##  Lower abdominals

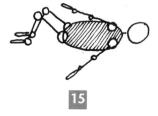 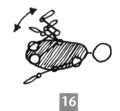

15. Bring your knees up towards your chest, forming a 90° angle, and then **16.** bring your knees towards your chest as you exhale. Return to starting position. Four sets of ten.

##  Thigh firmer

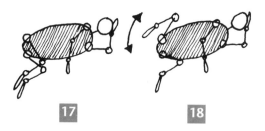

17. Lie on your side, with both knees bent at hip-level, as if you are sitting in a chair. Bend your elbow and support your head on your arm.

18. Lift your upper leg straight up, with your knee bent, bring it down, lift it up again. Four sets of ten. Repeat other side.

## Inner thighs and hip flexors

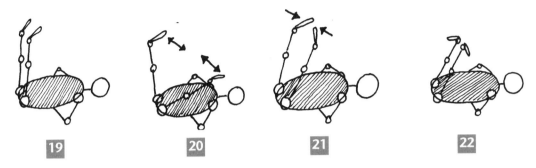

**19. 20.** Lie on your back with one hand on top of the other under the small of your back. Raise both legs straight up and bring them together and out ten times.

**21.** Do the same thing, but this time make your toes touch each other, ten times and then

**22.** touch your heels together ten times.

## Buttocks and pelvic floor muscles

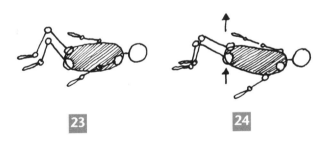

**23.** Lie on your back, knees bent, feet on the floor.

**24.** Lift pelvis and at the same time squeeze your buttocks together, also squeezing the internal, pelvic floor muscles. Do four sets of ten.

Stretching

Count *slowly* to twenty as you hold the stretch with every movement. Breathe in and out *slowly* as well to help you relax.

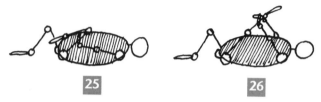

25.  Still lying on your back with one knee bent and your foot on the floor, hug your other knee to your chest and hold for a count of twenty.

26.  Raise this leg straight up towards the ceiling and hold with both hands for a count of twenty. Repeat with other leg.

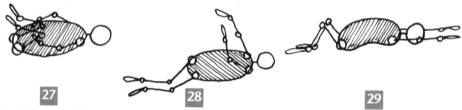

27.  Bring both knees into your chest, hold them there with your hands for a count of twenty, and then, **28.** bring both knees to the left and the arms to the right, hold again in the same way. Repeat on other side.

29.  Put your feet on the floor, knees bent, stretch your arms behind your head, and carefully arch your back to stretch the abdominal muscles.

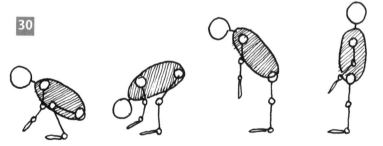

30.  To finish, get up on hands and knees, then on your feet, and with knees bent, roll up your back slowly, until you are standing straight.

You have finished the programme, don't you feel good?